Praise for *The Body Ecology Guide to Growing Younger*

"A few years ago I attended a weeklong workshop with Donna Gates. It was an eye-opening experience, as she shared simple but powerful principles for attaining and maintaining a superhealthy body. One of the most important things in the workshop. Donna fed us breakfast and lunch. We were able to taste and experience how delicious the fermented foods were. Everyone enjoyed her way of cooking and was delighted to take her recipes and probiotic nutrition home with them. I have been a follower ever since, and at 84 am enjoying vibrant health. Thank you, Donna Gates."

— **Louise L. Hay,** *New York Times* best-selling author of *You Can Heal Your Life* and co-author of *You Can Create an Exceptional Life*

"I love this book! Our national health has become an emergency, and Donna Gates provides the solution. . . . Scientifically and clinically based, this book provides a user-friendly, comprehensive handbook for our care and feeding into healthy longevity. Read it and stay young."

— **Hyla Cass, M.D.,** author of *8 Weeks to Vibrant Health*

"Donna Gates packs every page of **The Body Ecology Guide to Growing Younger** with health principles and nutrition advice that help rejuvenate your life and allow you to actually grow younger based on the latest breakthrough natural health technologies. This inspiring book empowers your healing, improves your life experience, and gives you tools to live over 100—all while having 'the best day ever' every single day!"

— **David Wolfe,** creator of The LongevityNOW Program; author of *Superfoods: The Food and Medicine of the Future, Eating for Beauty,* and *Amazing Grace*

"Donna Gates has always been on the cutting edge of nutrition and wellness. She is a vibrant example of the profound anti-aging potential of nutrient-dense living foods. I urge anyone who is interested in living a long and vibrant life to follow the principles contained in **The Body Ecology Guide to Growing Younger.**"

— **Jordan Rubin,** founder of Garden of Life; *New York Times* best-selling author of *The Maker's Diet*

THE
BODY
ECOLOGY
GUIDE TO
GROWING
YOUNGER

ALSO BY DONNA GATES

THE BODY ECOLOGY DIET: Recovering Your Health and Rebuilding Your Immunity (with Linda Schatz)

HAY HOUSE TITLES OF RELATED INTEREST

YOU CAN HEAL YOUR LIFE, the movie, starring Louise L. Hay & Friends
(available as a 1-DVD program and an expanded 2-DVD set)
Watch the trailer at: **www.LouiseHayMovie.com**

THE SHIFT, the movie, starring Dr. Wayne W. Dyer
(available as a 1-DVD program and an expanded 2-DVD set)
Watch the trailer at: **www.DyerMovie.com**

*THE BEAUTY BLUEPRINT: 8 Steps to Building the Life
and Look of Your Dreams,* by Michelle Phillips

*GREAT SEX, NATURALLY: Every Woman's Guide to Enhancing
Her Sexuality Through the Secrets of Natural Medicine,*
by Dr. Laurie Steelsmith and Alex Steelsmith

THE HEART OF THE MATTER: Gifts in Strange Wrapping Paper,
by Dr. Darren R. Weissman and Cate Montana, M.A.
(available September 2013)

*MEALS THAT HEAL INFLAMMATION: Embrace Healthy Living
and Eliminate Pain, One Meal at a Time,* by Julie Daniluk, R.H.N.

YOU CAN CREATE AN EXCEPTIONAL LIFE,
by Louise L. Hay and Cheryl Richardson

All of the above are available at your local bookstore,
or may be ordered by visiting:

Hay House UK: **www.hayhouse.co.uk**
Hay House USA: **www.hayhouse.com**®
Hay House Australia: **www.hayhouse.com.au**
Hay House South Africa: **www.hayhouse.co.za**
Hay House India: **www.hayhouse.co.in**

THE
BODY
ECOLOGY
GUIDE TO
GROWING
YOUNGER

Anti-ageing Wisdom
for Every Generation

DONNA GATES

(The bestselling author of *The Body Ecology Diet*)
with Lyndi Schrecengost
Featuring Body Ecology Medical Advisor Leonard Smith, MD

First published and distributed in the United Kingdom by:
Hay House UK Ltd, 292B Kensal Rd, London W10 5BE. Tel.: (44) 20 8962 1230; Fax: (44) 20 8962 1239. www.hayhouse.co.uk

Published and distributed in the United States of America by:
Hay House, Inc., PO Box 5100, Carlsbad, CA 92018-5100. Tel.: (1) 760 431 7695 or (800) 654 5126; Fax: (1) 760 431 6948 or (800) 650 5115. www.hayhouse.com

Published and distributed in Australia by:
Hay House Australia Ltd, 18/36 Ralph St, Alexandria NSW 2015. Tel.: (61) 2 9669 4299; Fax: (61) 2 9669 4144. www.hayhouse.com.au

Published and distributed in the Republic of South Africa by:
Hay House SA (Pty), Ltd, PO Box 990, Witkoppen 2068. Tel./Fax: (27) 11 467 8904. www.hayhouse.co.za

Published and distributed in India by:
Hay House Publishers India, Muskaan Complex, Plot No.3, B-2, Vasant Kunj, New Delhi – 110 070. Tel.: (91) 11 4176 1620; Fax: (91) 11 4176 1630. www.hayhouse.co.in

Distributed in Canada by:
Raincoast, 9050 Shaughnessy St, Vancouver, BC V6P 6E5. Tel.: (1) 604 323 7100; Fax: (1) 604 323 2600

Cover design and typesetting: John T. Davidson: jrocket77@mac.com
Interior design: Tricia Breidenthal

The hardcover edition of this book was published under the title *The Baby Boomer Diet: Body Ecology's Guide to Growing Younger* (ISBN: 978-1-4019-3545-0).

The Body Ecology Diet™ is a trademarked term.

A catalogue record for this book is available from the British Library.

ISBN 978-1-78180-144-4

Printed and bound in Great Britain by TJ International Ltd.

*This book is dedicated to my delightful,
charming, and very wise granddaughter,
Mia, and to the billions of children who will
be born generations from now. You inspire
me to do the work I do and motivate me
to want to live a long, healthy life and
be here to see the amazing world
you will create upon this earth.*

*My prayer is that this book will spark
the baby-boomer generation and our
children, your parents, into action
and create for you an opportunity
to inherit strong physical bodies and
brilliant minds that are in harmony
with your already-radiant souls.*

CONTENTS

PART III: Anti-Aging Therapies for Everyone

FOREWORD

I have known Donna Gates for nearly a decade. During this time we have worked together with many families who have children with serious conditions, including autism and autism spectrum disorders. I have watched her tirelessly and selflessly work for these kids and their families, teaching them about the foods and methods of her Body Ecology program.

My background is in gastrointestinal surgery and health, and Donna and I have often consulted together to find the best ways to communicate the principles and advantages of Body Ecology to multiple audiences, particularly to health practitioners who are seeking to understand the medical underpinnings of the program and share it with their patients.

Donna and I have lectured and conducted several seminars together on the principles of Body Ecology for physicians, other healthcare professionals, and the lay public, as well as for students planning a career as Body Ecology consultants. At some point, we became aware that this program would be a solid foundation for most anyone dealing with any type of illness, and that it would be particularly beneficial for people who are beginning to experience some of the effects and possibly the health concerns associated with aging.

The Body Ecology program includes eating whole, organic foods, either raw or cooked gently so as to maximize the nutrient content. In addition, there is a strong emphasis on fermented foods, while eliminating simple sugars. Such a program will balance and heal the gut lining, optimize gut flora, and minimize intestinal candida, thereby promoting good intestinal health. Today, science has shown that many conditions such as arthritis, allergies, autoimmunity, and neuroinflammatory ailments, as well as several forms of cancer, have significant connections to an unhealthy intestinal tract. Throughout this book, you will see how the Body Ecology program also confronts many of the diseases and concerns of aging, from cosmetic issues such as wrinkles to more serious health problems, such as Alzheimer's.

I was pleased to be asked to serve as the medical consultant on this project, and was eager to share my perspective on the benefits and applications of the Body Ecology program as seen through the eyes of someone intimately involved in health and wellness, and who has witnessed the power of this program firsthand.

— **Leonard Smith, M.D.**
Medical advisor to Donna Gates & Body Ecology

PREFACE

We live on an amazing planet. What new, undiscovered worlds wait to entice us? A tranquil lake in the Canadian Rockies? A painting on a wall of the Louvre? A smile of recognition on our new grandchild's face? Will we have the chance to enjoy these "mountaintop experiences," or will time run out for us?

What if we knew in advance what our final years would look like? Can we imagine a day when we are too frail to drive our cars? Can we imagine a time when we can no longer recognize a place we've been to a thousand times before, or can no longer hear our granddaughter's sweet voice? Can we imagine not doing all the things we've worked our whole lives to be able to do? The great irony of aging is that we may finally have everything we need materially, but no longer be able to enjoy it and share it with those we love most.

Despite the current statistics and the common belief telling us we are living longer, healthier lives, it is clear that something isn't right. Degenerative conditions such as heart disease, cancer, diabetes, obesity, osteoporosis, and stroke are causes of serious concern for all of us. Aging itself is a degenerative disease. Fading vitality, wrinkles, sagging skin, obesity, gray hair or no hair, and diminished sex drive are just a few of the symptoms of an unhealthy body. The signs of aging begin long before we are "old," but they often go unnoticed. Aging happens quietly and cunningly, and it speeds up with time, startling us with abrupt and dramatic changes that weren't there yesterday but are here today.

Statistics suggest that many of us will suffer from heart disease, cancer, diabetes, obesity, osteoporosis, and/or stroke. Unlike our parents, who accepted these diseases as unavoidable, today's generations know that there must be another way. As a result, we are taking interest in new forms of health-care technology, drawn from both traditional and complementary medicine. We are also rediscovering precious ancient knowledge to empower us to achieve the health we so strongly desire.

The Body Ecology program is part of this new vision—an advance in how to resolve the problems of aging and disease. No other system of wellness is as balanced or as complete. As health educators, my team of Body Ecologists and I have been on the front lines of some of the most challenging issues facing people today, from autism to obesity to immunological disorders. Because we work every day with real people with real problems, we are intimately aware of emerging health trends and concerns.

The foundation for Body Ecology is food—what to eat, in which combinations, and how to prepare it. The effect of food on the body cannot be underestimated: how we feed ourselves is not just about satiating hunger; it's about creating a healthy inner ecosystem that supports a vibrant and active life. The basics of the Body Ecology food program are outlined in detail in my first book, *The Body Ecology Diet*. Many of the principles developed in that book are also part of an effective anti-aging program, and will be covered in Parts I and II of *The Body Ecology Guide to Growing Younger*. In addition to how we eat, however, there are lifestyle changes all of us can make, easily and quickly, to reverse the signs of aging and increase longevity. Many of those important choices will be carefully covered in Part III.

The "Body Ecology Way of Life" is not my creation. Around our offices we always say that you can see "the hand of God" in this work. This knowledge is here because it's time. It's time for us to understand the missing pieces that create *genuine* health. We age because of ignorance, because of choice, and because we live in a world that supports early aging and degenerative conditions. Since its inception, Body Ecology has had the mission to change ignorance to understanding when it comes to the way we eat and care for our bodies. We exist to be a catalyst for creating a paradigm shift toward the true science of health and healing in this world—a paradigm shift that will benefit our children, grandchildren, and great-grandchildren for generations to come.

— **Donna Gates**

PART I

A NEW WAY OF LIFE

CHAPTER 1

FOREVER YOUNG:
An Introduction to the Body Ecology Way of Life

*Armed with knowledge, medical evolution, and
the power of our own minds and wills, we can literally
transform how we live the next phase of our lives—
as well as the legacy we leave future generations.*

Consider this: had you been born in the late 1800s, your life expectancy would have been about 45. Today, that doesn't seem like nearly enough time to live a full life. It seems inconceivable that, had we lived little more than a century ago, life might almost be over at the age of 40.

We've come so far! It is a brilliant time to be alive, because there is so much more that we now know about how to stay young and healthy. Today we are privileged to reap the benefits of medical breakthroughs—and also holistic and nutritional advances—that make agelessness not just conceivable, but a *reality*. We will live longer than any previous generation, and we have the *potential* to live better—with the opportunity to reinvent what it means to be in our "golden years."

And yet, something is not quite right. In his book *The Hundred-Year Lie: How Food and Medicine Are Destroying Your Health,* journalist Randall Fitzgerald notes how many middle-aged people are afflicted with diseases that used to be reserved for "old age"—from multiple sclerosis to cancer to Parkinson's and Crohn's disease. The petro-chemical era of the 20th century initiated an onslaught of toxins that are exacting a heavy price on this and subsequent generations. As Fitzgerald notes, between 1952 and 1987, the production and use of synthetic pesticides in the U.S. increased 13 times faster than before the Second World War.[1] From genetically modified foods to sex hormones, from industrial contaminants that pollute our air and water, to overuse of antibiotics and inoculations, seemingly inescapable toxins have besieged our bodies for decades.

Environmental toxins alter our DNA. They damage our immune systems. They increase our predisposition to illness and disease. And they are passed on, through the umbilical cord and blood of the mother, to our children and grandchildren. In fact, from the moment sperm and egg cells come together, toxins are already present. Children born today are coming into the world with serious infections, weakened immune systems, and increased susceptibilities to certain diseases.

In addition to the accumulation of toxins in our bodies, we grapple with new psychological stresses as we age. Rising life expectancy, aging parents, and faulty pension plans mean that many of us will need to work much longer than our parents did, whether we want to or not. This makes our continued good health not wishful thinking but a practical necessity.

As we struggle to stay young, many of us have turned to quick-fix solutions—cosmetic procedures, anti-aging hormones, and extreme diets—to stave off the aging process. But these methods are akin to repainting a dilapidated car. At first glance, these cosmetic changes may improve the appearance, but they don't account for more important and deep-seated issues. These can only be addressed through an understanding of our inner ecosystem; and how diet, food purity and selection, and lifestyle choices can lessen the effects of aging, giving us not just *longer* lives, but *better* ones. That is what this book is about.

How Body Ecology Came to Be

My own healing and happiness evolved out of a very personal health crisis and recovery. I was born with a sensitive constitution. It seemed as a child I was always coming down with lung infections and suffering stomachaches, and many of the foods I ate didn't agree with me. When I was 15, my skin began to break out, and a well-meaning but misguided dermatologist prescribed antibiotics. Fifteen years later, frequent use of antibiotics had weakened my body to the point where I had almost no functional immune system, and my stomach burned whenever I ate anything. By the time I was 30, I could tolerate only about five foods.

This launched me on a personal quest; and I began to explore every kind of diet available, including vegetarian, raw, macro, natural hygiene, and high protein. I also spent a fortune on supplements and found real value in neuromuscular massage, acupuncture, colonics, and craniosacral therapy. Everything helped, but I still felt weak, and my digestion never improved.

At the age of 38, confused and uncertain as to where to turn next, I found that fate intervened. I met Dr. William Crook, who had just written *The Yeast Connection.* After reading his book, I realized that I had a classic case of an extremely common systemic infection called *candidiasis.* The infection and its toxins had seriously compromised my digestive, immune, and endocrine systems.

After much study and trial and error, I eventually created an entire system of health and healing centered around repairing and restoring my inner ecosystem—killing off the bad yeast and the accompanying viruses and then recolonizing my intestines with friendly microbiota, thus restoring proper digestion. I called this system "Body Ecology."

More than anything else, I am a teacher, so naturally I began to share what I was learning with others. I knew my discoveries needed to reach more people, and in 1994, I published the first edition of *The Body Ecology Diet*—a program designed to help others heal their own inner ecosystems through dietary and lifestyle changes. Slowly the book made its way around the world to the people who needed it. I also founded a nutrition company called Body Ecology, Inc.

Two decades later, the system of healing I was guided to create is providing answers to many other health challenges—including the problems associated with aging. Unbelievably, *The Body Ecology Diet* is currently in its 11th edition and is now published by Hay House. It has helped tens of thousands of people return to optimal health. I can see so clearly the happier, healthier, younger world that is possible through the Body Ecology Way of Life.

What Is the Body Ecology Way of Life?

While Body Ecology has evolved into a way of life, it began as a diet. Our digestive systems are intimately linked to our immune, endocrine, circulatory, and central nervous systems. A healthy digestive ecosystem—which I will talk about much more later in this book—is the first step toward a long and vibrant life. In the same way, most if not all of the signs of aging can be ultimately connected back to the way we eat—how we allow toxins to build up in our bodies, and how effectively we eliminate them from our systems.

But the Body Ecology Way of Life also includes lifestyle choices that go beyond diet. By learning how to honor the gifts we were given at birth—including our relationship to the sun, our breathing, our connection to the earth, and more—we are able to foster well-being and increase longevity naturally and effectively. For this reason the first two parts of *The Body Ecology Guide to Growing Younger* will focus on the healthiest approach to food and diet, but in Part III we'll cover effective and sometimes unexpected anti-aging therapies that support maximum health at any age. Together, these approaches form the "Body Ecology Way of Life."

It Starts with Our Thoughts

From the Body Ecology point of view, growing younger starts with our thoughts. Our thoughts and emotions are always reassembling and reorganizing, but they follow our instructions! We can transform our reality if we change our beliefs. In fact, the body acts like a puppet to our thoughts, and it has a tremendous capacity for self-healing *if* we focus on health, not disease.

My friend Louise Hay, the founder of Hay House (the publisher of this book), is a wonderful example of how thinking "different" can change the future. I first met Louise when she attended a Body Ecologist workshop. I was quickly inspired by her balanced way of taking care of her own growth and needs while helping the world and seeking the truth. Her openness and availability to new ideas keeps her perennially young and engaging. She follows the Body Ecology Way of Life, and it is wonderful to see how her body and demeanor are in harmony with her youthful spirit. Louise is a great inspiration to me, and a powerful model for those who may think getting older means limitations rather than opportunities.

Have you been resigned to or obsessing over the changes in your body? If this continues to be your focus, you will certainly find more and more signs of aging with each passing year. Instead, I encourage you to begin—right this moment—to direct your thoughts to how it looks and feels to be young. Focus on what you want to *become,* not on what you currently *are.* Your body will begin to respond with new health and vitality.

Now, imagine if all of us collectively start to concentrate our thoughts on how it looks and feels to be young. Our cells will respond immediately, and the universe will begin to give us what we want. Why would it do this? Because the universe wants this, too! If millions of us remain young and healthy, we can be of much greater service to the world. We can begin the work we have come here to do.

It is my greatest hope that this book will become the first in a series of "inspired thoughts" that will guide you toward a younger, healthier, and even happier you.

CHAPTER 2

WHY WE AGE:
Finding the Fountain of Youth Within

*Armed with new knowledge about what accelerates
aging and disease, we can transform the way
we view, experience, and treat getting older.*

From the 16th-century explorer Ponce de León, who believed he'd found the waters of agelessness in Florida, to the myth of Shangri-la, a paradise where aging does not exist—we humans have long sought the Fountain of Youth. Have you, too, ever wished that you possessed the secret of eternal youth? I certainly have. Wouldn't it be wonderful if it were as simple as a magical elixir or potion . . . or perhaps the perfect antiwrinkle cream?

There are many theories on aging. Each offers valuable insights into the role that food, nutrition, and lifestyle play in longevity. Understanding *why* we age will give us the knowledge we need to *prevent* aging and, just as important, to *reverse* existing signs of aging.

Theories of Aging

Before we learn how to halt the aging process and grow younger, it's important to understand why we grow old. Here are some of the more popular theories being discussed today—ending with Body Ecology's own theory on aging.

— The **genetic** or **DNA theory of aging** argues that we were born with a blueprint encoded within our DNA that predetermines our physical and mental weaknesses and strengths, and regulates the rate at which we age. By far the most well known of all the theories, it is also sometimes referred to as the *planned-obsolescence theory* . . . a rather depressing idea, isn't it? The good news is that DNA can be positively or negatively affected by diet, toxins, lifestyle, environment, and even our thoughts. In other words, our choices—past, present, and future—can accelerate DNA damage or slow it down. The reins are in our hands.

— The **free-radical theory of aging**, developed in the 1950s, maintains that aging is due to the accumulation of free radicals— very small molecules that have lost an electron, become unstable, and then attack the closest stable molecule, stealing its electron. The attacked molecule becomes a free radical, and a domino effect starts, resulting in the deaths of many cells.

Free radicals are a natural by-product of life. They form when you breathe, eat and burn glucose for energy, detoxify dangerous chemicals, are injured, or do strenuous exercise. But if you have a poor diet, drink too much alcohol, smoke tobacco, are under chronic stress, are exposed to radiation, and/or push yourself too hard when you exercise, you are accelerating your body's production of free radi- cals—and the "oxidative damage" they cause.

Healthy cells can overcome minor attacks from free radicals, but when those attacks become more intense, and there are not enough antioxidants in your body, your cells begin to die—speeding up the aging of the body and brain, perhaps even causing premature death. Free radicals create waste products that interfere with DNA, RNA, and protein synthesis; cause inflammation; lower your energy levels; and generally disturb vital chemical processes throughout the body. In short, they accelerate aging, and one of the most obvious signs of their handiwork is wrinkles. Fortunately, there are many antioxidant- rich foods, herbs, and supplements (especially the fermented foods and probiotic liquids) available that you can consume every day to help combat the damage of free radicals.

— The **inflammation theory of aging** has received a lot of press of late. Integrative physician Mark Hyman defines inflammation as "the activation of the immune system due to the presence of some kind of intruder," such as an infection (viral, fungal, or bacterial), allergen (mold or ragweed, for instance), or toxin (heavy metals, pesticides, and xenoestrogens). This inflammation can be obvious, such as eczema or psoriasis, or it can be subtle, working deep inside us at the cellular level (for example, inflammation of the arteries, leading to heart disease).[1]

When we don't eat properly, fail to hydrate or get enough sleep, allow ourselves to become overweight, are overcome by stress or besieged by environmental toxins, or avoid sunlight and become deficient in vitamin D, we increase inflammation in the body.

While inflammation makes us more susceptible to aging, aging in turn makes us more susceptible to inflammation. To break free from this vicious cycle, we must balance our immune system and build a hardier one to conquer the infection. To trigger a "youthening" in our cells, we must cleanse our cells of toxins, balance our hormones, and nourish them properly. *A gluten-free, sugar-free probiotic diet can cool the fires of inflammation,* reducing tissue breakdown.

I tend to view inflammation as both a symptom and a cause of aging. While a poor diet is certainly a major cause of inflammation, a nutrient-rich one can become your most important tool to reverse it.

— The **hormonal-decline theory of aging** (also called the *neuroendrocrine theory of aging*) involves diminishing levels of critical hormones. Our hormones are secreted by little organs or glands— the hypothalamus, pituitary, thyroid, adrenals, ovaries, testes, pineal gland, and pancreas. As we age, we become more toxic and malnourished, and these glands lose their ability to secrete their respective hormones. In addition to this dramatic decline in production, our trillions of cells lose their sensitivity and will no longer "accept the hormones," even if the body is still making them or getting them from an outside source.

As this decline occurs, cortisol and insulin become elevated in our blood. These two hormones work together as a team; as cortisol levels climb and remain high, so do blood sugar and insulin. The excess sugar and insulin permeates our bloodstream, causing weight gain, elevated blood pressure, and unremitting acidity of bodily fluids. An acidic environment is the perfect home for infections and cancer. Low levels of sexual hormones and elevated insulin are hallmarks of early aging.

— The **mitochondrial-decline theory of aging** suggests that augmenting and protecting our mitochondria is an essential part of preventing and slowing aging. The mitochondria are organelles (tiny organs) found in every cell in the body. They are powerful energy generators, using oxygen and glucose to create the fuel that every cell needs.

Unique to the mitochondria is that they have their own DNA. But this is actually a problem in terms of aging. While other kinds of DNA have histone proteins and repair enzymes to protect them, mitochondrial DNA does not, which means the mitochondria are subject to greater free-radical damage. The mitochondria become larger, more tired, less efficient, and fewer in number as we age.[2]

The primary job of the mitochondria is to create energy (*adenosine triphosphate,* or ATP). Having enough energy is essential for the repair and regeneration of every cell inside your body. Very little ATP can be stored in the body; our reserves are quite small. Thus, the mitochondria have to be efficient and healthy in order to produce the continuous supply of ATP we need.[3] The decline in ATP production and loss of mitochondrial efficiency can lead to diseases such as cancer.[4]

But mitochondria play an even greater role in longevity than we once knew. A recent study conducted at Harvard Medical School and published in *The Journal of Molecular Evolution* has revealed that our mitochondria are of paramount importance in prolonging life span. These scientists discovered that mitochondria are not static and unchanging; they have actually evolved over time in a way that has "allowed humans to lead longer, healthier lives without the scourge of neurodegenerative disease."[5] As mitochondria are now being viewed as central to the evolution of human longevity, it is important to explore proven methods for supporting and enhancing these organelles.

— Related to the mitochondrial-decline theory is the **glycation theory of aging.** Glycation can reduce the functionality and efficiency of mitochondrial proteins, which in turn promotes cell death. Glycation takes place when the body's proteins or DNA molecules bond chemically with sugar molecules, eventually forming rogue molecules called *advanced glycation end-products* (AGEs). AGEs in tissues increase free-radical production to many, many times the rate produced by unglycated proteins, which has been associated with accelerated aging. We create AGEs in our bodies when we cook our foods, especially our animal protein, at high temperatures. We also create them by allowing our blood sugar to become elevated. Those of us who have insulin resistance or diabetes are constantly creating AGEs.

Glycation plays a role in a wide range of problems, including cardiovascular disease, stroke, cataracts, arthritis, and atherosclerosis.[6,7] AGEs also trigger inflammatory reactions throughout the body, including the brain, where they have been shown to cause certain cells to pump out free radicals that are toxic to neurons. Many scientists believe that AGEs play a significant role in cognitive-decline diseases such as Alzheimer's.[8]

— There are two additional cell-related theories of aging. First is the **cell-membrane theory of aging**—which suggests that as we grow older, the cell membrane becomes less lipidic (watery), inhibiting cell functioning and leading to accumulation of toxins. The second is the **Hayflick limit theory of aging,** which suggests that a human cell can divide only a limited number of times. Dr. Leonard Hayflick theorized that a cell divides approximately 50 times, after which it dies. Hayflick's research showed that we can slow down the rate of cell division through the right diet and a healthy lifestyle. In particular, he found that calorie restriction might play a role, as underfed cells divide much more slowly than overfed ones.[9] (See Chapter 6.)

— The **Body Ecology theory of aging** is really very simple. The two principal causes of aging are: (1) an accumulation of toxins in our cells, and (2) nutritional deficiencies in our cells. Both of these factors weaken our cells, resulting in a loss of our core energy and vitality, leading to degenerative disease, including aging. The information in this book will help you reverse both of these processes—not just to halt the aging process, but to actually help you grow younger.

The Chinese Medicine Theory of Aging

It is interesting—but not surprising—that in every theory of aging, lifestyle and diet have a clear and dramatic impact, whether negative or positive. This is also true of the Chinese medicine theory of aging, which offers its own unique insights into aging and how to do it more gracefully. I've highlighted this theory of aging because it is one we at Body Ecology embrace—and it factors into how we can create more youthfulness and longevity in our lives every day.

In the West, we live in a youth-obsessed culture. We admire the beauty and vitality of younger people, and we don't want to admit that we may have lost our own. People in the Far East have a very different attitude toward aging. They focus on the quality and vitality of life at any age . . . how to live long, happily, and full of youthful *energy.* They believe that the essence of aging is not in how we *look,* but in how we *live.*

Remember, what you focus on is what you get. You don't want to focus on aging; you want to put all your thoughts and intentions into *creating youthfulness.*

Ancient Chinese medicine understood that we age when our energy wanes and eventually becomes depleted, causing us to become vulnerable to what Western doctors call "disease." Body Ecology avoids the term *disease,* preferring the more positive Eastern concept of *imbalances,* as this model is more empowering. If something is out of balance, the obvious solution is to put it back *into* balance.

Why is there an imbalance? Do you have an infection? Is your digestion weak and your body lacking in vital nutrients? Are you deficient in most hormones but have too much insulin circulating in your blood? Are there toxins in your system that are dampening down your life force? If yes, then you have it within your own power to address and correct these imbalances.

Let's take a closer look at energy—the vital life force. Where does it come from? How do we get more, and how do we keep our energy balanced?

Jing Energy: A Gift from Our Ancestors

In Chinese medicine our primal energy comes from the inherited prenatal life force we had before we entered this world *(jing)* and from the energy we acquire as we nourish our bodies day by day *(chi)*.

Were you born with a strong constitution? Was your fundamental intrinsic energy once quite strong? This is the result of jing energy (or essence energy)—the prenatal, primordial energy given to us from our parents, grandparents, and ancestors. If our mothers ate well and had a happy, easy pregnancy with very little stress; and if our ancestors were strong, hardy people, then we would have inherited strong jing energy.

More than anything else, constitutional energy determines longevity and controls the aging process and our resistance to disease. Strong jing generates a long life that is free of degenerative disease. Weak jing shows itself as a failure to thrive (in children) and premature aging (in adults). It determines our ability to rejuvenate. Our sexual vitality and how "sexy" we look and feel is directly related to our prenatal energy.

If our parents did not understand how important it was to eat well, to cleanse their bodies of toxins, and to reduce stress in their lives—both prior to conception and while our physical bodies were being formed—then we were, in truth, victims of the ignorant times into which we were born.

Although our jing energy is fixed and inherited, it can be conserved by our actions throughout the day. Because it is *stored* energy, it provides the reserves we need to adapt to all the various toxins and stresses we encounter in modern life. Jing energy can be steadily depleted as the years go by. For some of us, it was depleted quickly because of our diet and lifestyle choices. If we learn to protect and even build up these inherited reserves, we can look and feel amazingly youthful even in our 50s, 60s, 70s, and beyond.

Imagine that each of us had a rich uncle, Freddie. Your "Uncle Freddie" gifted you with $5 million on the day you were born. (You inherited a really strong constitution.) *My* Uncle Freddie may have only had $2 million to give to me. (My parents were not as healthy as yours.) Let's pretend that from the moment we were born, you and I began to spend our money. You spent yours faster than I did mine because you had more than I did, but even so, by the time we were both in our 50s, we were broke. Our constitutional energy was depleted, and we could actually feel that it was.

But my friend Sara, who, like me, only received $2 million, was taught to never draw money from her account unless she also put much of it right back in. Sara led a busy life, too, but she never ate sugar, and loved fermented foods and vegetables. She also exercised moderately and managed her stress through yoga and meditation. Not surprisingly, when she reached 50, she still had most of her inherited money. As a result, she looked and felt 20 years younger than we did.

Jing is exactly like this. If each day we spend what we've inherited and never replace it, we will reach our older years looking and feeling pretty spent.

You must make *daily* investments into the inherited account so that you have something to draw upon in times of added stress and demand. If you know that the day ahead calls for a lot of energy, you will want to fuel your body with those foods, herbs, and supplements that give you that needed extra energy (see the explanation of chi to follow) to get you through that day.

We drain our accounts when we smoke, drink alcohol and coffee, or eat a diet of refined foods that contain a lot of sugar and poor-quality fats. Add stress, poor sleeping habits, overwork, too little exercise, and a poor understanding of how to conserve our sexual vitality, and we have a perfect description of most of the aging population. Even chronic and acute illnesses deplete jing. Diminished sexual desire, weight gain, memory loss, graying hair, sagging skin, and poor muscle tone should be seen as evidence that we've "misplaced" (not lost) this essence of rejuvenation. Sadly, we have taught this way of life to our children, who are now teaching it to our grandchildren.

Chi Energy: A Gift from Ourselves

Chi (sometimes spelled "qi") energy is *acquired* energy. It is our daily life force—it powers us to move and to thrive. It suffuses every living thing; resides within every cell, organ, and tissue; and affects every stage of our growth, from conception to death. When we are healthy, the body is a fountain of constantly circulating chi—a lovely dance of yin and yang that nurtures a sense of balance, harmony, and wellness.

Chi energy is the key to maintenance of health and the prevention of disease. After birth, chi comes from the good things we take into our bodies, along with their proper digestion and transformation. It is the energy we obtain day after day as we feed ourselves nourishing foods. These nutrient-rich fruits, vegetables, herbs and roots, proteins, fats, and seeds have a life force of their own and contribute to our reserves.

Some foods have no nutritional power unless they are altered in some way to make them easier to digest. In fact, there is an art to preparing foods in a way that increases their life force so that they, in turn, increase *ours*. As humans, we have the ability to change the nature of foods by cooking them, fermenting them, and sprouting them to enhance their inherent life force. Many have to be prepared to make them more digestible so that we can "get the most out of them."

As infants—and even as older children—we had very little ability to obtain our acquired chi on a daily basis. Even if our mothers offered us healthier foods, did we really want them? After all, most kids are happy with sweet-tasting, lifeless foods. As adults, we find that these items have become embedded in our cellular memory, and they are now our comfort foods in times of stress.

Chi energy is created through our daily choices. But even before we can focus on our chi, there's another kind of energy that must be in place. To live a long and happy life, we must first invest in the energy that in Chinese medicine is called *shen,* or spiritual energy.

Shen Energy: A Gift from Our Creator

Chinese masters say that *shen* is an all-embracing love that expresses itself in our hearts. It presides over the emotions and communicates itself outwardly as an all-encompassing compassion, acceptance, and tolerance toward others. Shen energy is our guiding spirit, a wonderful manifestation of our higher nature as humans. When our "shen is off," we are dispirited, brought low by life's stresses, toxins, and traumas. But when we are "full of shen," we dare to live to the fullest! When our intrinsic prenatal energy is restored and meets with the energy in our hearts, our shen energy can open outward so that we act from a place of forgiveness and unconditional love. Amazing changes can be accomplished almost immediately.

Strong shen is essential for well-being; it gives us our willpower. Without it, restoring our prenatal jing and creating daily chi are difficult to achieve. In turn, the interaction of jing and chi leads to vital shen. When shen, jing, and chi are in perfect balance, our minds are strong, our emotions are balanced, and our bodies are vital and healthy.

Jing, Chi, and Shen—the Three Treasures

Constitutional energy (jing), daily acquired energy (chi), and spiritual energy (shen) are together called the three heavenly treasures. They are gifts for us to cherish as we live upon this earth in our physical bodies.

Besides the three heavenly treasures, we have been given earthly treasures as well. All over the planet, humankind has been provided with countless wonderful foods, herbs, air, water, and an amazing variety of life experiences with which to nourish ourselves. The 7 Principles of Body Ecology—and the food groups you will discover in this book—will provide you with the foundation you need to sort through the limitless possibilities.

Replenishing Our Youthful Energy

Many of us look in the mirror and see that we have not done a very good job of nourishing ourselves. Much of our core intrinsic energy has dissipated, and we don't know how to replenish it. We aren't even aware of how to acquire energy day by day. Each one of us must now ask: "What can I do to restore my depleted *inherited energy?*"

The answer: For each remaining day of your life, you must begin to create—step by step—enough energy to carry you through the day, *plus extra* to replenish the prenatal energy that has been exhausted from a lifetime of neglect and a lack of knowledge. Whether it is out of fear of becoming old and suffering the pain of aging, or out of vanity because we do not like what we see in the mirror, many of us are ready to take this action. The action we must take is to follow the Body Ecology Way of Life.

The rest of this book will provide you with the valuable tools you need to do just this—and to reverse the signs of aging and rejuvenate your jing and chi in the process. It all starts with cultivating the "inner garden," which we'll discuss in the next chapter.

From the Physician's Desk

"It isn't what you eat that ages you. It's what
happens to what you eat that ages you."

One theory is that aging is due to chronic low-grade systemic inflammation that the body is not managing efficiently. The Body Ecology system is an ideal anti-aging strategy because it manages inflammation through appropriate diet. But Body Ecology is not just about food. The Body Ecology system is about eating the right kinds of food the right way, *and making other lifestyle choices that support a healthy inner ecosystem*. Ultimately we want to heal the gut lining so that the life-giving attributes of food have the opportunity to get through and do their best work.

Along with the right foods eaten the right way, it's important to find methods for detoxifying and decompressing the stress in your life. Drinking lots of water, ridding the body of toxic metal poisons using infrared saunas, habitual exercise that sweats the toxins out, regular sleep, and work that fulfills you and makes you happy are simple but tried-and-true methods of managing stress and giving your inner ecosystem the greatest chance of thriving.

— *Leonard Smith, M.D.*

CHAPTER 3

THE MISSING PIECE:
A Healthy Inner Ecosystem

Within each of us is a miraculous inner ecosystem.
Most of us are ignorant of its existence at all, yet
it is essential to our health, immunity, and longevity.

We've explored the vast reaches of space; the dark depths of the ocean; the intricate workings of the brain; and even the beautiful, once-invisible, world of the womb. There is, however, a microscopic universe within our own bodies that has, until now, been by and large uncharted and unknown. It is the last, perhaps *greatest,* frontier. At Body Ecology, we call this unexplored secret world the "Missing Piece"—the single most important building block for health, immunity, and, certainly, longevity.

This Missing Piece is our inner ecosystem . . . the intestinal garden that is established deep inside our belly as we leave the womb. Visible only with a microscope, it is a delicate inner world, and it requires perfect balance and harmony for us to flourish.

As the term *inner ecosystem* is largely unknown, I've created a definition that describes the ideal, healthy inner ecosystem we should all strive to attain:

A healthy inner ecosystem is a dynamic "garden" of beneficial and neutral bacteria and yeast that are also called microbiota. They live and associate with their environment (your intestines), creating a vibrant interrelating community. These energetic microbiota are surrounded by your enteric nervous system or "gut brain" (sometimes called your second brain); and are related to the transfer of energy and materials into your nervous system, your brain, and the rest of your body.

The inner ecosystem is so vital to your well-being that as you continue to read this book, you might soon be asking yourself, "How have I overlooked the importance of my own inner garden?"

The word *garden* originates from an old German term, *gart,* meaning "enclosure." A garden can be as simple as a pot of herbs in your kitchen, or it could be as vast as the rain forest in South America, rumored to be an ancient garden from another era. For many, the garden is a sacred space—a place of spiritual connections.

An ancient Chinese proverb says: "If you want to be *happy* all your life, plant a garden." But I'd like to add: "If you want to be *healthy* all your life and *live a longer one,* cultivate and fertilize your sacred *inner* garden."

Body Ecology teaches that the garden inside us should be lovingly tended and respected as sacred. With careful husbandry, it will protect us from dangerous diseases and the physical effects of aging.

Nature's Secrets Revealed

Humans, fish, birds, and even insects—in fact, all living animals— have an *inner ecosystem in their intestines.*

Unlike plants, which are rooted firmly in soil, animals are in constant movement. We do not stay in one place and, therefore, must carry our "soil" inside our own bodies. A tree acquires its nutrients from the soil in which it was planted, but we humans carry ours around with us *in our gut.* If that precious soil is depleted and stressed, we may develop the human equivalent of root rot, fungal infections, spotty leaves, and so forth. Or we may just fail to thrive and prematurely die.

When you were in the womb, if your mother ate a nutritious diet rich in fermented foods, and if she had strong constitutional *jing* energy, you would have been well nourished during your growth and development. Beneficial microbes would have naturally colonized *in your mother's digestive tract* and *in her birth canal* so that when you entered the world, your own pristine intestines would be *immunized* with the "good little bugs." You would now be able to safely eat and digest your next food: mother's milk.

The natural sugars found in your mother's breast milk would soon stimulate the growth of these indispensable microbiota, and in just a few months, this thriving inner world of beneficial beings would be working together to protect and support you so that you could live safely in the outer world. These microbes would help your body digest nutrients; neutralize toxins; metabolize vitamins; balance hormones; and keep pathogens such as fungi, yeast, and parasites in check.

Sadly, since this was an unheard-of phenomenon (and mostly still is), many of us were deprived of this sound foundation. In fact, by the middle of the last century, breast-feeding had fallen out of favor. Few people understood the life-giving properties of mother's milk. Breast-feeding was considered inconvenient—even embarrassing— and many fathers were uncomfortable with it.

Paradise Lost

Some of us may have been fortunate enough to have enlightened parents who understood the importance of creating a toxin-free, nutrient-rich environment within the womb. But most of us were not that lucky. The wonderful prenatal energy that should be the rightful inheritance of every child was denied us—and now our children and grandchildren.

Before our birth, our mothers ideally should have eaten ferment-ed foods and liquids. That would inoculated the birth canal with healthy bacteria and yeast so that when we emerged from the womb, we would have quickly developed a strong, hardy immune system that would allow us to live in a world that contained pathogenic mi-crobes. We would have also digested our foods properly and would have healthy intestines, blood, and cells. We would not crave refined, sugary foods and would be satisfied with the natural sweetness in fruits and vegetables.

Body Ecology views the inner and outer ecosystems as parallel. We all know what happens to the atmosphere, to our water supply, and to our food when environmental pollutants are not kept in check. Our toxic planet becomes inflamed, fatigued, and unbalanced. In the same way, without beneficial microbiota present in our inner world to help keep us clean inside, we are literally walking about with polluted bodies that *cannot* detoxify naturally, in spite of our best efforts.

Let's return to our soil metaphor . . . fertile soil is *living* soil, containing billions of microorganisms. Today we have no memory of a time when farmers practiced ecological farming—planting different crops every year and rotating them so that the balance in the soil was preserved—but it used to be the rule. Instead of using chemical fertilizers, these "eco-farmers" enriched their fields with manure, putting organic matter back into the soil to reenter the ecological cycle.

Today, farming is controlled mostly by the petrochemical industry, which has had a disastrous effect on the quality of our food and our health. Fritjof Capra, author of the famous book *The Turning Point,* refers to synthetic fertilization as "agricultural chemotherapy," which depletes the humus content in the soil and affects a crop's ability to take up and absorb nutrients.[1] Depleted, overused, and compromised with fertilizers and pesticides, this dry, "dead" soil is more susceptible to wind and water erosion and produces food that has a fraction of the nutritional value it is supposed to have. You cannot expect healthy food to come from wasted ground. In the same way, you cannot expect to enjoy radiant health when your own internal "biological terrain" is weak, stressed, and defenseless.

By replenishing our own inner gardens—the complex and dynamic ecosystems inside our gut—we create an environment that sustains us, driving our health and protecting against disease and the typical assaults of aging.

Finding Our Youthful Secret Garden

I have often wondered why the secret—the "Missing Piece"—has remained hidden from us for so long. I've come to believe that we have finally advanced far enough in our spiritual awareness that we are now asking the right questions of our Creator . . . and receiving the answers. We have recognized the great achievements of modern medicine, but we've also seen its limitations. More and more of us are realizing that all of the state-of-the-art medical advances and technologies in the world will avail us nothing if we've lost our connection with the earth that sustains us. The Missing Piece asks us to reestablish this vital connection, intended for us at conception, but now seemingly lost.

When you build your Body Ecology, you are creating a living, thriving inner ecosystem that supports your health—doing all the work of creating energy and longevity on the inside of your body. Wouldn't it be ironic if the legendary "Fountain of Youth" was not a source of water at all, but rather a "secret inner garden" that holds the key to youthfulness? While water is certainly essential for life and longevity, perhaps igniting our digestive *fire* is just as important.

In the previous chapter, you learned how *shen, jing,* and *chi* are critical to health, and how the latter in particular is related to what we take into our bodies. Chi is dependent upon what Taoists call "digestive fire," the ability of the stomach and spleen to "ripen" food, transform it, and turn it into energy. Many foods in the standard American diet, with its emphasis on processed sugars and flours, "dampen" and slow down this digestive fire.

The Body Ecology approach encourages balanced but diverse methods of food preparation—from lightly steaming and low-temperature sautéing and baking to raw foods and even fermenting. These, and the powerhouse foods themselves, will ignite your digestive fire, not only delivering more nutrients, but also making them more "bioavailable" (accessed and used more effectively). And, unlike any other way of eating you may have tried before now, the Body Ecology Way of Life honors and helps create your amazing inner garden, bringing life, vitality, and youthfulness back into the power center of your body: your intestines.

Louis Pasteur's Legacy

More than 100 years ago, Louis Pasteur, a French microbiologist, proposed a new theory of disease called the "germ theory." It continues to exert a powerful influence on medicine to this day. Peering through his microscope at a sample of spoiled wine, Pasteur observed a colony of active "little unseen bodies" (germs), and determined that if the growth of these germs, or what he called *microorganisms,* was the cause of the spoiled wine, it could just as well be the cause of contagious disease. In Pasteur's mind, these microorganisms were "bad," and it was necessary to prevent them from entering the body.

Pasteur's ideas about germs were partly true. We know that bad, or unfriendly, bacteria and viruses feed and multiply, causing the body to become susceptible to infection, fatigue, and degenerative disease. Pasteur's work led to the development of antiseptic surgical methods that ultimately saved countless lives—in fact, until doctors began washing their hands before delivering babies, one in three women died in childbirth.

Pasteur's efforts and discoveries were truly revolutionary, but they were also myopic. He noticed that the little bugs inside the wine were easily destroyed when the wine was heated. From that point on, medicine took on a troubling bias—that disease was caused by outside, invading forces that made victims of us all. It was this largely fear-based germ theory that also led to pasteurization; mass immunization; and, eventually, the discovery of antibiotics.[2]

Working against nature rather than with it has led to the present state of affairs in medicine today. In fact, Pasteur stated in his acceptance speech to the French Academy of Sciences that the experimenter is one who tries continually to conquer nature.[3] Pasteur had a very limited understanding of one of the most important universal laws of nature—the *Principle of Balance* (which will be discussed in greater detail in Chapter 4). Indeed, he forgot to point out that the successfully fermented wine contained good "little unseen bodies." We live in a world of opposites. There is a positive and negative side to everything, including bacteria. Pasteur left out a vital part of the truth.

Here are just a few of the many reasons why beneficial microbiota must be present in the gut for us to be healthy:

- **Beneficial microbiota ensure that we are well nourished,** and help eliminate nutritional deficiencies that cause our bodies to fail and age quickly.

- **They assist in the breakdown of foods.** By acting as enzymes, these bacteria support the digestive process.

- **They produce vitamins.** The B vitamins, vitamin K, and biotin are produced deep inside of us, where they can enter immediately into the body.

- **They help extract and retain minerals from our foods.**

- **They prevent toxins from causing damage to the intestinal lining.** This damage leads to disorders such as irritable bowel syndrome, Crohn's disease, and colitis.

- **They protect us against colon cancer.** Ingestion of viable probiotics and prebiotics—food that nourishes beneficial bacteria—is associated with anticarcinogenic effects, one mechanism of which is the detoxification of genotoxins (agents that damage DNA) in the gut.

- **They are essential for immunity.** The mechanisms by which probiotic bacteria affect the immune system are not yet fully known, but many microbiota are correlated with an increase in the innate or acquired immune response. In fact, 70 to 80 percent of our immune system is located in the gut, where microbes are critical for protection against disease.

A hundred years later we are suffering from this one-sided view of nature. Sadly, we have created an entire system of healing called "modern medicine," which is not a system of healing at all. It is a disease-management system based on fear and focused on killing "bad bugs," viruses, and cancer cells with drugs, surgery, and radiation. Modern medicine, with its emphasis on killing and cutting, instead of building the positive forces in nature, has taken many lives it might have saved. Iatrogenic disease (a health threat caused by doctors and medicines) is within the top ten causes of death in the U.S. According to a study of 37 million patient records by HealthGrades, a health-care quality-assessment company, an average of 195,000 people in the U.S. died due to potentially preventable, in-hospital medical errors in each of the years 2000, 2001, and 2002.[4] And they haven't solved the problem yet. Hospitals are dangerous places full of dangerous microbes.

To a great degree, Pasteur's discoveries led to as many problems as they solved. If only he had noted that the superb wines of France contained beneficial bacteria and yeast, as did sourdough breads, cheeses, and sour-milk products (kefir and yogurt)—and if only he had promoted the benefits of an environment where the good bugs not only ruled but also destroyed the bad bugs—we might be living in a very different world today.

Another Side to the Story

Some of Pasteur's colleagues at the time argued that the *environment* of the blood surrounding the cells was the cause of disease—not the bugs. They believed that something in the environment of the wine allowed the bad bugs to flourish. They were adamant that something happening within the body and blood was allowing pathogenic bacteria, viruses, fungi, and cancer cells to grow. As you will soon learn when you read about the *Principle of Acid and Alkaline* in Chapter 4, Pasteur's colleagues were correct.

A century later, we are beginning to see the negative consequences of Pasteur's "all or nothing" approach to bacteria. Pasteur believed that a healthy body had no bacteria in it.[5] In our society we've been taught to be afraid of bacteria. Bacteria mean "germs." It is a nasty word to many of us, evoking the source of disease and sickness. In truth, however, we live in a world where good and bad exist together, and this is certainly the case in the amazing world of microbiota.

In his zeal to eliminate pathogenic bacteria from the world, Pasteur made an unfortunate mistake. His method of pasteurization, developed to prevent milk from spoiling, also prevents it from fermenting into "clabbered" milk (milk that sours and thickens naturally). Because it ferments naturally, clabbered milk contains a much higher number of healthy microbes and is far better for you than just raw milk. Pasteurization, by contrast, robs milk of some of its most life-giving nutrients and destroys naturally occurring friendly flora that cause it to safely ferment.

Why did this mistake occur? Why were people not allowed to know the complete truth? Perhaps it was simply a matter of timing. Perhaps we could not appreciate truth until we had made a devastating blunder first. We humans do tend to learn best from our own mistakes. By experimenting with killing, cutting, and radiating our way to health, we are now ready for another, wiser path to wellness.

In a nutshell: If you focus on the positive, creating a world inside your body of cooperative, constructive, and supporting beneficial microbes, then health, happiness, and longevity will follow.

Microbiota—Warriors on the Intestinal Battlefield

Medical science's 100-year error has provided us with a unique perspective on what we want—and what we do not want. Now our thoughts and intentions can reach out for a better way. Body Ecology offers that "Missing Piece" that Pasteur and the rest of the world didn't see—a radical (but long-overdue) way of looking at beneficial microbiota, the foods that contain them, and the role they play in our digestive tracts and in keeping us young and healthy. Hidden *deep inside each of us,* they mean the difference between surviving and *thriving*—they are the key to unlocking a longer, healthier, and happier life.

The Missing Piece is the foundation of the Body Ecology program for growing younger, since understanding the need for a vital inner ecosystem is the first step toward the health we are all hoping for. The next step, however, is to understand the 7 Universal Principles of Body Ecology—seven guidelines that will help you make the right choices in what you eat and how you live. These principles will be covered in the next chapter.

From the Physician's Desk

"All diseases lead to the gastrointestinal tract."

Julius Caesar famously said, "All roads lead to Rome." When it comes to disease, one might say, "All diseases lead to the gastrointestinal tract." This would appear to be the case, as so many medical conditions we see today are largely due to intestinal issues. Poor-quality food—which is not digested properly—is sending the wrong information to the intestinal lining, resulting in inflammation and increased intestinal permeability. The resulting "leaky gut" allows for more absorption of unwanted food substances, microbial toxins, and bacteria themselves . . . all of which cause the immune system to become imbalanced.

When this happens, your immune cells may produce antibodies that affect body parts such as the joints and pancreas—contributing to arthritis and type 1 autoimmune diabetes, as well as many other conditions. The medical term for this phenomenon is *antigen mimicry,* where antibodies that are being produced to ward against food and toxins "cross-react" and attack normal human tissues. This is just one of many mechanisms whereby damage to the gut lining, with increased permeability, may lead to systemic diseases.

— *Leonard Smith, M.D.*

THE 7 UNIVERSAL PRINCIPLES OF BODY ECOLOGY

Food—and how it is prepared and eaten—is the foundation of the Body Ecology Way of Life. But how do we know what foods to eat—and in what combinations? The 7 Universal Principles answer these questions for us.

Body Ecology's 7 Universal Principles are guidelines for eating and healing. These are universal principles or laws that all of nature and all humans must obey. Together they weave a system that flawlessly supports our health and longevity. Used correctly, they can guide us to the answers and solutions to prevent and even reverse the symptoms of aging. They teach us how to increase our vitality and well-being for years to come.

In the pages that follow, I offer you an overview of each of these principles—just a taste, to help you understand where the dietary elements of the Body Ecology anti-aging program come from. A much more in-depth look at each of these principles can be found in *The Body Ecology Diet*.

The Principle of Uniqueness: Knowing Yourself

The first of the 7 Universal Principles, the *Principle of Uniqueness* states that you are a singular, one-of-a-kind individual. That's it: you're *unique.* Yes, we have most of the same pieces and parts: a heart that beats, lungs that breathe, eyes that see, and a brain that thinks. But we have diverging needs; childhood experiences; habits; and ways of thinking, learning, and being. These differences give us identity and individuality. Your uniqueness will bring its own properties to the Body Ecology program; and the Body Ecology Way of Life is flexible, so it can be altered somewhat to meet your special needs.

The journey begins with honest self-evaluation: where are you, right now, today; and how prepared are you to embark on this new program? The first step is to get a clear snapshot of your current health status. By visiting your holistically oriented doctor (one trained in functional medicine), you can obtain helpful tests such as a hormone panel and a genetic profile and check the status of your minerals, fatty acids, and amino acids. You can find out what heavy metals are in your body and even determine your biological age (versus your chronological age)—all of which will help clarify your unique needs.

The Principle of Step by Step: Knowing Where and How to Begin

The Principle of Step by Step is the universal law that tells us that we can't do everything we would like to do or need to do all at once. If we try, we will surely fail. Learning and change do not happen overnight. We must face them step by step. By the time you have finished reading this book, you will have learned many new tools to help you reverse aging. But please, don't try to pick up all of them right away. You can't. Take a minute to tune in to your intuition, and notice which steps feel most urgent and appealing. Try those first. Master one or two, and then add another when you are ready to do so.

You have most likely heard the expression that "a journey of a thousand miles begins with the first step." Here are four simple steps you can take in *your* journey toward reaching the Fountain of Youth. They will help you maintain or regain your youthful energy and appearance.

1. Create Energy

First and foremost, create energy. Nothing else can happen until this initial step has been taken. Most of us begin experiencing loss of our prenatal *jing* energy by our 30s. It may first manifest itself in joint and muscle pain or a general feeling of life seeming kind of flat.

But there are other signs. Do you feel spacey and forgetful at times? Suffer hormonal imbalances? Are you losing muscle tone? Often constipated? Are you no longer sleeping well? These are just some of the many symptoms that show that your vital prenatal jing and your daily chi energy have been compromised.

To prevent or reverse aging, you must maintain or restore your original *jing*. Many of us must be particularly mindful of this, especially if we are overachievers, stay very busy, and tend to feel that we aren't really "living" unless we're "doing." We've never learned how to relax. Too many things compete for our time and our energy—the Internet, cell phones, television—filling our world with incessant chatter. We may not even be aware of how much the static has increased over the years. To slow down aging and rejuvenate, we must begin to learn how to conserve our energy and find ways to nourish ourselves.

Take a few moments to consider the things that are draining you of vital energy: Not enough sleep? Too many commitments? Toxic relationships? The amazing superfoods and anti-aging therapies found later in this book will provide you with excellent solutions to begin renewing your energy day after day . . . step by step.

2. Conquer Infections

During the course of your lifetime thus far, how many different drugs have you taken? Vaccinated often as children and given frequent rounds of antibiotics, we are the first generations to reap the rewards but also suffer the devastating effects of pharmaceutical-driven medical care. Alcohol and recreational drugs play an important role in our social life, and we have so much sugar abundantly available whenever we want it.

Well, today eight out of ten Americans suffer from candidiasis. The drugs, alcohol, stress, and sweet foods so available to us have accelerated this yeast/fungal problem (which you are most likely experiencing right now). The lifestyle we lead gives fungi even more opportunity to thrive. This serious chronic infection becomes more acute as our immunity diminishes with age, and this sets the stage for cancer.

The Body Ecology system of health and healing, with its amazing "Diet," originally began as a way to conquer yeast infections. It is the most complete and comprehensive antifungal diet available. The Diet and its 7 Principles are just as effective for preventing and reversing aging as well. Infections cause inflammation, which then causes us to age. Diagnosing and conquering all infections is essential to any anti-aging program.

When infections like candida are corrected through the Body Ecology approach, energy automatically goes up, and susceptibility to disease goes down. Other common infections most of us are struggling with include viral herpes; bacterial infections in the gums; low-grade, chronic bacterial infections in the bladder; and *H. pylori* bacterial infection in the stomach, causing ulcers.

These all deplete the body of energy. When they are conquered, the energy to rejuvenate and to stay young becomes yours.

3. Correct Digestion

When the digestive tract doesn't work well, nothing works well. Are you experiencing some of the signs of a compromised digestive tract, such as constipation, diarrhea, inflammation in the gut, irritable bowel syndrome, and flatulence? It is essential that you heal your gut lining and establish a healthy inner ecosystem, repopulating the intestinal tract with friendly microbiota.

Body Ecology has an excellent understanding of gut health and provides us with valuable tools for having a healthy digestive tract throughout life. When first starting The Diet, during the first five to ten days, many people with an inflamed mucosal lining will want to "rest" the gut by eating primarily soft or liquid foods—broths, purees, and green smoothies—and also lightly steamed leafy-green and ocean vegetables.

4. Cleanse from Toxins

We must actively remove the toxins from our bodies. These toxins are in our organs and in our cells. They come to us from nutritionally deficient, poorly digested, and poorly combined foods. They are in the water, in the air, and even in our self-destructive feelings. They are in drug residues and ingested metals, such as lead, aluminum, and cadmium. We have inherited toxins from our parents, and we pass them on to our own children. Toxins snuff out our spiritual power and our intuition. When they are removed from our lives, boundless energy is created. Doing so is essential for young men and women who want to have beautiful, healthy children. (See more on cleansing later in the chapter.)

Making Progress

Taking a step-by-step approach to healing doesn't mean that your progress has to be slow. You can choose how quickly you embrace the steps, and you may experience immediate improvements in energy and vitality. On the other hand, you might need to go at a more moderate pace. Be realistic. Don't take on more than you can handle. When you feel comfortable with one step, move on to another.

Here are four simple steps you can take in the beginning that can make an enormous difference in your goal to regain your youthful energy and appearance:

1. Cut back on or eliminate sugar and high-carb sweets. Even those so-called energy bars are loaded with sugar, depleting your essential prenatal life force. Instead, you will be introduced to several alternative sweeteners that will allow you to still enjoy the sweet taste without the

damaging and aging effects of sugars . . . even honey and the "healthy" sugars.

2. Change the oils you are currently eating to the extra-virgin, unrefined fats and oils of The Diet. Later in this book you'll be provided with a delicious array of fats and oils to keep you looking and feeling great. They also make eating more pleasurable.

3. Add some fermented foods to your diet, such as fermented vegetables and young coconut kefir. This is perhaps the most important step of all, as you'll soon learn.

4. Pay attention to cleansing your colon. You might consider trying your first colonic, if you've never had one before (see Chapter 19). Cells must eliminate their toxic waste. When you're constipated, so are your cells. They, too, feel toxic, sluggish, and irritable. Actively cleansing with diet, herbs, colonics, and home enemas will soon become commonplace as more of us begin to understand that we must purify our bodies to maintain and reclaim our youth.

Success comes step by step. That's why you must be very determined to stick with The Diet until you master it. Advance according to your own personal pace, but persevere. As you begin to implement The Diet, I hope you will treat your body as an evolving experiment in self-awareness. Unlike other dietary approaches, the Body Ecology Way is not a short-term "fix," but rather an ongoing journey of personal discovery and adaptation.

The Principle of Cleansing: Purify from the Inside Out

I've briefly mentioned cleansing in the preceding section, but this is also one of the 7 Universal Principles. In fact, nature is always cleansing herself with wind, rain, heat, and snow. Cleansing is nature's way of allowing the body to get rid of unwanted toxins, waste, and foreign substances, playing a vital role in preventing disease and aging.

If we are to remain forever young, toxins must come out of the cells in our organs. Cleansing is the process that accomplishes this—carrying away cellular debris. If we had or still have strong prenatal *jing,* we will also have a strong ability to cleanse.

Many of the signs and symptoms of aging are a direct result of the vast amounts of toxins we've accumulated since conception. They are stored in the liver, causing it to be congested; our joints ache, our skin wrinkles, and our eyes develop macular degeneration. Toxins devastate our sensitive endocrine system, which produces anti-aging hormones, such as HGH, melatonin, DHEA, progesterone, and testosterone. When we peel back the layers of this mostly unintentional damage, we begin to feel, and certainly look, years younger.

What most of us don't realize is that our bodies are constantly working on our behalf to purify and cleanse us of these toxins. Aging cells are constantly being replaced with new ones. A speck of dust gets in your eye, and you blink and tear up—to cleanse out the dust so it won't hurt you. A similar thing happens when a virus invades your system and you get a fever; it's your immune system working to purify your body of that toxin. In fact, the ability to purge toxins out of each cell is really quite remarkable. (We pay extra for ovens that are self-cleaning, yet our bodies do it for us for free!)

But over time, our cleansing organs begin to wear down. For example, the liver—that miraculous and overburdened organ of detoxification—shrinks as we age. By the age of 70, it will likely have decreased to 81 percent of its original size. It will not only receive a smaller blood supply, but it will also be less able to do its important job of cleansing. If we choose to use drugs, they will no longer be eliminated as efficiently, predisposing many of us to overdose. A better solution is to follow the recommendations for foods, supplements, and cleansing therapies in The Diet . . . fermented foods, healthy fats, enzymes, and colon cleansing.

When we're young, our cells have walls that are soft and pliable. As the body begins to fill with more and more free radicals, these walls, made of a fatty membrane, become hardened. (To get a better idea of what happens to your cells as you age, place a lemon on the counter and watch how the skin hardens from the oxygen.)

If cell walls remain soft and pliable (from antioxidant-rich plant foods), nutrients carried in your bloodstream enter your cells, while waste products are sent back out into the bloodstream, where they are eliminated in a variety of ways. Examples of how the body eliminates toxins are: bowel movements, urination, skin eruptions, sweating from a fever or the summer heat, tears, vomiting, coughing up mucus, and (special to women) the monthly menstrual "cleansing."

Unfortunately, we have been taught that cleansings are "bad" and need to be suppressed, so we pop a few pills, keep on working, and try to pretend they're not really happening to us. Indeed, while we were growing up, we were brainwashed to stop the cleansing.

Our Bodies Were Created to Remain Young!

As we get closer to death, we will begin to lose the ability to purify unless we choose (with strong intention) to change this natural course of events and actively help our bodies cleanse with diet, herbs, home enemas, colonic therapy, saunas, chelation, and other therapies described in this book.

If you had or still have strong prenatal jing, you will also have a strong ability to cleanse. One of the secrets to remaining forever young is to never lose this ability to purge toxins and waste. Instead, welcome—and assist your body in—this natural process.

As you better understand the Principle of Cleansing, you will feel both the gratitude and joy that comes with realizing that our bodies were created with this amazing function embedded within us—this ability to purify in order to heal and stay young.

The Principle of Balance: The Dance of Yin and Yang

The Principle of Balance focuses on the balance between *yin* and *yang*, contractive and expansive energy. Yin and yang are complementary opposites, two interdependent and creative forces of change that are always seeking equilibrium.

Yang energy is outward, activating, drying, and warm or hot. It may stimulate thoughts of the sun and of fire. Yin energy is inward, stored energy. It is nourishing, moistening, cooling, and anti-inflammatory. It may remind you of water or of the moon.

Since illness and disease are caused by imbalances, we must pay close attention to whether yin or yang dominates in the body. Yang illness emerges when there is too much fire energy (inflammation) or when we are too stressed-out (uptight, with pulses racing). Yin illness occurs when we are too depleted (fragile, exhausted, and anxious).

As we age, we have traditionally become too yin (weak and depleted). This weakness allows inflammation (too much heat or yang energy) to thrive in our bodies. The right foods and supplements help us build the foundation to reverse the signs and symptoms of aging.

Remember, one of the primary anti-aging goals of Body Ecology is to create more *daily chi energy* and to restore our *prenatal jing energy*. Both can be accumulated or stored for later use, or exhausted or used up entirely. The foods on the Body Ecology program create the foundation we need to balance, rejuvenate, and store energy.

The Principle of Acid and Alkaline: How to Choose Your Foods

One of the most amazing features of the human body is its ability to keep its internal state relatively constant. The pH—or balance between acid and alkaline—of our blood, saliva, and urine is carefully regulated within a narrow range. The ideal pH of blood should be 7.36 to 7.44; if it drops below 7.2, it has become dangerously acidic and we can die. An even *slightly acidic decline* in pH, however, allows infections and disease and even cancer to develop inside us. It's vital that we maintain our blood close to the ideal of 7.4, especially if we want to reverse and prevent aging.

If you feel that you're aging too quickly, you must pay special attention to this Principle of Acid and Alkaline. Indeed, one of the main reasons why we age is because the body becomes acidic. To keep your body more alkaline, your diet should consist of foods mostly from the plant kingdom—especially vegetables from the land and the sea. The more color, the better: dark green, leafy vegetables and dark—even black—ocean veggies, properly prepared so that you can digest them, are excellent examples of alkaline foods that keep your body within that ideal pH range.

Eighty percent of your food intake should be these alkaline-forming foods, which will be outlined fully in Part II of this book.

The Principle of Food Combining & the Principle of 80/20: How to Eat

The last two principles—Food Combining and 80/20—both have to do with optimizing your digestion. Many of the diseases that cause aging begin with poor digestion. Fortunately for us, these two principles—along with fermented foods, discussed in Chapter 6—can take the burden of having to work so hard to digest your meals off your digestive tract.

Food combining means to deliberately eat certain foods with other foods. We do this because simply combined meals, where the foods digest easily together, obviously allow the stomach, small intestine, and colon to do their job more efficiently. As a result, nutrients are more accessible. There is less bloating and gas in your digestive tract, and also less inflammation. Incompatible foods that do not digest properly ferment and cause an overproduction of sugars, foul-smelling stools, diarrhea, and constipation. This also creates more toxins and more acidity in your body.

Food combining often seems complicated to people, yet it is actually one of the easiest of the principles to implement. In fact, if you practice it for one week, it will become second nature to you. There are six simple rules to food combining:

- **Rule #1:** Eat animal protein with non-starchy vegetables.

- **Rule #2:** Eat grains and grain-like seeds (that is, quinoa, millet, buckwheat, and amaranth) with starchy and non-starchy vegetables.

- **Rule #3:** Eat fruit alone and at least 30 minutes before any other meal, or combined with a protein/fat (see Rule #5). Or eat acidic fruit combined with leafy-green salads.

- **Rule #4:** Combine fats and oils with animal protein, grains, grain-like seeds, and starchy or non-starchy vegetables. Basically they go with everything.

- **Rule #5:** Combine protein/fats with other protein/fats. (Protein/fats are foods that contain both protein and fat, such as avocado, dairy foods, and nuts and seeds.)

- **Rule #6:** Combine protein/starches with non-starchy vegetables from the land and ocean. (Protein/starches, such as beans, contain mostly starch but also a small amount of protein.)

While these basic rules will get you started, there is much more to learn about food combining. If you are interested in expanding your understanding, this principle is covered at length in *The Body Ecology Diet*.

The Principle of 80/20 works well in conjunction with that of Food Combining, as both are about correcting and improving digestion. Many of us have "eyes that are bigger than our stomachs." We eat huge portions, consuming not only to the point of satiation, but usually well beyond that. This puts far too much stress on our already-overtaxed digestive tracts. The 80/20 Principle prevents this issue with three simple rules:

1. **Eat until your stomach is 80 percent full, leaving 20 percent available for digestion.** This means leaving the table before your stomach is full. You can always come back and eat more later!

2. **Eighty percent of the food on your plate should be land and/or ocean vegetables, with the remaining 20 percent reserved for a meat protein, a grain, or starchy vegetables.** Vegetables are the staple of the Body Ecology Way of Life. Fill 80 percent your plate with non-starchy varieties, and with this alkalizing, high-fiber diet, you'll live a longer, healthier life.

3. **Approximately 80 percent of the foods on your plate should be alkaline forming, and 20 percent should be acid forming.** This rule counteracts the American tendency to eat a preponderance of acid-forming foods—animal proteins, breads, cereals, pasta, and starchy vegetables. Non-starchy vegetables are key to creating an alkaline environment in your body. A body that remains more alkaline retains more minerals—key nutrients for beauty as well as longevity.

You can read much more about the 80/20 Principle—and all of the principles outlined in this chapter—in *The Body Ecology Diet*. But for now, this baseline understanding of the principles will allow you to better "digest" the information coming up in Part II—the section where you'll get the specifics you need in order to begin cultivating your inner garden, and staying young the Body Ecology way: from the inside out.

SUPERFOODS THAT CREATE A YOUNGER YOU

CHAPTER 5

THE ART OF EATING

*Most of us completely underestimate the power of food.
Foods are far more effective in restoring energy and modulating
oxidative stress than any supplement or drug on the market today.
Along with our positive thoughts and intentions, food offers
us the greatest potential to reverse the aging process.*

Most of us completely underestimate the power of food. To obtain the most possible nourishment from our food, we must not only know what to eat, we must also know *how* we eat it. So even before we get into the details of the delicious foods and simple preparations that make up the dietary component of the Body Ecology anti-aging program, we will start here: how to eat in such a way that our food nourishes our souls. Then, we can move on to discuss the properties of Body Ecology foods—foods that nature has given us to heal the body and keep ourselves young throughout the decades.

Food as Energy

Food affects us emotionally and spiritually. It has an intrinsic energy and intelligence that it communicates to us on a cellular level (see sidebar on page 47). This energy can actually alter our behavior, performance, and appearance. I've seen many lives elevated—renewed and healed—through the power of wholesome, nutritious food.

Because of its healing potential and spiritual energy, food should be sacred to us—prepared with reverence and consumed with gratitude. But alas, even though the passing decades have brought us more insight and wisdom, many of us still make our food choices based on our taste buds and our desire for immediate gratification.

Every time we eat, we must now be asking ourselves, "What does my body *need*, not just *want?* How can I nourish and heal myself with the food I put on my plate today?"

As we make our eating choices, it is wise to also reflect on how the food was grown or raised, how it was slaughtered and transported to us, and so forth. These choices not only impact us on an individual level, but have global implications as well.

Most of us today will remain quite active and busy as the decades pass. We will still need plenty of energizing nutrients (protein, minerals, vitamins, antioxidants, enzymes, and small amounts of high-quality fats and oils) to sustain our dynamic lifestyles. But because our bodies won't be as efficient at digesting foods, we will need to learn ways of preparing them so that we can utilize their nutrients more effectively.

Eating *less* and eating *foods of higher nutrient density* are two of our most important tools for keeping youthful, disease free, and fit. We should bring positive thoughts and intentions to *how* we eat as well; and mealtimes can be wonderful opportunities to practice developing our hearts, minds, and wills.

Our Very Cells Recognize Food as Friend or Foe

Every piece of food we consume comes into contact with our cell surfaces, which are loaded with receptors that identify it as positive, neutral, or negative. Our cells recognize something as a "friendly food" or an "unfriendly food." There is a whole field of science devoted to this, called *nutrigenomics,* or the way food as information speaks to our genes. Food elements contact cell surface receptors, which pass the information to cell messengers called *kinases, chemokines,* and *cytokines.* These messengers take the information to the nucleus and give it to the genes. This process is called *signal transduction.*

Our genes respond positively to organic, natural foods—in other words, a mostly plant-based diet, including properly prepared grain-like seeds, land and ocean vegetables, fermented foods, and a modest amount of organic animal products. The genes in our cells respond positively when they receive messages from a simple piece of broccoli, containing myriad health-giving molecules with names like *indoles, carotenoids, lutein, glucosinolates, isothiocyanates, sulforaphanes,* and many more.

Mindful Eating

In his book *The Yoga of Nutrition,* Omraam Mikkael Aivanhov, a spiritual master from France, writes: "Food is a love letter sent to us by our Creator, and we must learn to read it. It is the most eloquent, the most potent of love letters, for it says, I love you and I am giving you life and strength."[1] Food is full of sunlight, flavor, color, shape, and texture. How sad that we swallow it without reading the love letter carefully.

Do you eat unconsciously or quickly so you can get on with the really important things in life? Instead of enjoying a meal quietly and consciously, are your daily cares and stresses churning about in your stomach? Do you leave the table feeling sluggish and sleepy?

It's little wonder many of us don't digest our foods properly. The *way* we eat is every bit as important as *what* we eat.

Many spiritual traditions practice mindful eating, which simply means to slow down and truly experience the aromas, flavors, and textures of the food. Chewing it slowly and well, and enjoying it in a quiet setting—rather than being rushed, agitated, and halfway out the door—is an essential part of this practice.

Part of the stress and anxiety so many of us feel today is because we have lost our connection with nature and our gratitude for her amazing gifts to us. When we eat with gratitude, we reestablish that vital link to the natural world around us. We must learn to have a deeper appreciation for those who make our meals possible; and, if we've prepared them ourselves, we do so with a listening spirit, allowing our intuition to take over so that we are tuned in to what our bodies are asking for in that moment. We come to learn the difference between eating until we are overfed and doing so until we are satisfied.

What else is involved in mindful eating? Preparing our meals deliberately and thoughtfully so that everything we need is easily at hand . . . setting a beautiful table . . . taking time to breathe deeply throughout the meal . . . designating a space and time that's quiet and uninterrupted—all these are ways we make eating a kind of spiritual practice, a sacred rite where food is transformed into strength, energy, love, and light.

Inside the Body Ecology Foods

So why have we chosen to highlight certain foods as part of your anti-aging arsenal? In other words, why do Body Ecology foods stand out?

- **Body Ecology foods are replete with fortifying *chi* energy**—ideal for anyone who wants to feel more vigorous and vital.

- **Body Ecology foods are *probiotic***—ideal for creating a strong, disease-free body. The word *probiotic* literally means "for life." Probiotics are living microorganisms that have a beneficial effect on the body because of the way they function in the digestive tract. Most probiotics contain *Lactobacillus* or *Bifidobacterium,* which are "good" bacteria. All of the anti-aging probiotic foods and supplements recommended here are safe, effective, and designed to enhance intestinal health.

- **Body Ecology foods offer a perfect balance of proteins, carbohydrates, and healthy fats**—ideal for people who have suffered through exclusionary, nutritionally lopsided diets.

- **Body Ecology foods are antifungal**—ideal for people with yeast infections.

- **Body Ecology foods are gluten and casein free**—ideal for people with allergies to wheat or milk protein.

- **Body Ecology foods are low in sugars**—ideal for people with weight issues, candida, or adrenal fatigue.

- **Body Ecology foods have the greatest bioavailability, meaning they are quickly and efficiently accessed by the body**—ideal for people with low energy and weakened digestive systems.

- **Body Ecology foods are nutrient-dense**—ideal for anyone who wants to look and feel better!

Some Things You Might Experience with Body Ecology Foods

New Tastes and Textures

Humans have six basic tastes—*sweet, salty, bitter, savory, pungent,* and *sour.* Probiotic foods provide the sour taste, which may be one that is less developed in you than the others. A wide variety of tastes and colors is essential to obtaining all the nutrients that food has to offer. Some of the Body Ecology fermented foods, such as young coconut kefir and milk kefir or cultured vegetables, may be a new taste sensation to you. Try to keep an open mind as you explore foods outside your comfort zone.

If at first you're a bit skittish about some of the foods, that's okay. Remember the Principle of Step by Step? It's okay to take your time. You'll soon find yourself choosing delicious grain-like seeds (like quinoa and millet) over pasta and rice, and adding sea vegetables to soups and stews and salads and stir-fries because you miss them when they're not there.

Over time your body has acquired a "memory" for the foods it thinks it wants, even if they are unhealthy! It will take a little time to "reeducate" your palate. After you've been eating the Body Ecology way for a few days, you'll begin to experience the more robust and potent flavors of pure, whole, well-combined ingredients. As your body acquires new food memories, the result will be a greater appreciation for the essence and aromas of truly healthy, satisfying foods. Time to reawaken your palate!

Intestinal Discomfort

If you're not accustomed to eating fermented foods, at first you could experience some indigestion (gas and bloating). This is because the mighty microbiota are busy changing their environment (your intestines) into a much more pleasant place. They want to survive, colonize, and thrive. In a week or so, this phase will pass; however, this is a good time to drink plenty of springwater (away from meals), make sure your bowels are eliminating well, and do enemas and colonics to cleanse yourself of the toxic material that is making you age way before your time.

Share What You're Learning!

I encourage you to experiment and explore! Find those foods that suit your tastes and needs the best. Getting to know these new foods and how to prepare them in fun and interesting ways is one of the joys of Body Ecology Way of Life. As a matter of fact, we welcome new recipes and discoveries. Please feel free to e-mail Body Ecology so we can share your recipe with others on our website: **recipes@ bodyecology.com.**

In the pages that follow, you will learn about new foods, new ways of preparing them, and how to maximize their benefits for optimal health and healing.

From the Physician's Desk

"Many of the foods we eat today are
new to our genetic code, and our genes
respond to them in often-negative ways."

For too long we have underestimated the impact of food on the body. Over the course of 70-plus years on the planet, our bodies take in 20 to 25 tons of food. The gut lining, like the lungs and the skin, is one of the most absorbent areas in the body, and as we know, three-quarters of the immune system is located there. Our greatest exposure to foreign material is through the food we eat, and this food provides critical information that is interpreted by the immune system.

The gut lining reads food like a book, and it recognizes what it likes and doesn't like, and whether the food is friend or foe. Food is not some undifferentiated substance that passes benignly through our systems and is never heard from again. It has qualitative differences. Until very recently, for example, we thought all protein was the same, whether in the form of beef, legumes, nuts, or fish. Now there's been a paradigm shift; and we know that just as with carbs, there are good, bad, and neutral proteins. We have finally begun to recognize that food consists not just of fat, protein, and carbohydrates, but of infinitely subtle messengers that communicate information to our bodies in profound ways.

Poor-quality food causes our cells to go into a defense mode and put our immune system on high alert. On the other hand, high-quality food—rich in antioxidants, enzymes, and minerals, with the right kinds of natural carbs that are slowly absorbed—speaks to our genetic code in a way that keeps our bodies healthy and happy.

— *Leonard Smith, M.D.*

CHAPTER 6

FERMENTED FOODS:
Anti-Aging Miracles

As ancient as the great Flood of Noah, fermented foods are becoming the new "stars" of the natural-foods world.

Modern science is now confirming that fermented foods are the quintessential anti-aging foods. They are essential to restoring our prenatal jing and are the true "superstars" of the natural-foods world. At Body Ecology, we are pleased to be able to teach you how to use them to reverse biological aging.

The focus on these ancient yet "new-to-you" foods is what makes the Body Ecology Way of Life stand out above all other "diets" being promoted today. It works! In fact, it makes the other ways of eating obsolete. This chapter shows you why you really *must* include fermented foods daily to regain the vitality of your youth.

What Are Fermented Foods?

By the middle of the last century, the refrigerator was an essential appliance in the home. Although we take it for granted, it is a relatively young technology. So how did people survive without refrigeration for thousands of years? They ate foods fresh from the fields and dried, smoked, and fermented them.

In some parts of the world, fermented foods are believed to be the food of Noah's ark, when the world was covered with water. They were certainly included in the diets of American Indians, who preserved their meats and fish by fermenting and smoking them. To ensure that they had vegetables through the long winter months, they fermented and then buried them in earthenware containers.

Probiotic-rich fermented foods may seem either foreign or familiar, depending upon your cultural heritage. All traditions still have their own versions of cultured foods, which are staples in the diet. In Germany, a significant percentage of fermented foods and beverages are consumed today in the form of beer, wine, sourdough breads, sauerkraut, kefir, and *kvass.* The Germans and Portuguese enjoy a regional raw, fermented sausage, called *rohwurst* and *chourico,* respectively.

In Russia, children are offered a glass of kefir (fermented milk) at school on a regular basis. In China, the government distributes cabbage to the population each fall to ferment and store through the cold winter months. Indonesians eat *tempeh,* a fermented soybean cake; and in Japan, fermented foods from both soybeans and dairy lead sales in the natural-foods arena, spurred on by a tremendous amount of research by doctors, food companies, universities, and medical schools.

Many of us grew up with cheese, sauerkraut, yogurt, soy sauce, and dill pickles—foods that are traditionally fermented. Unfortunately, the mass-produced versions found in our supermarkets are not probiotic. If you read the labels on these items, you'll notice that most are pasteurized and contain refined vinegar and poor-quality salt. Pasteurization by high heat destroys precious enzymes and beneficial microbes, and the addition of refined salt has contributed to many of the health problems we face today. These products are nothing like the live, enzyme- and microbiota-rich fermented foods and beverages we at Body Ecology encourage you to eat and drink each day.

Benefits of Fermented Foods

As we age, our nutritional requirements do not change, but the number of calories we consume should be reduced, especially once we're in our 40s.

Limiting the amount of food you eat per day—practicing calorie restriction while optimizing nutrition—is the one sure way that researchers agree slows and even reverses biological aging.

Moreover, it is a fact that you can't effectively or safely practice calorie restriction with optimal nutrition without having fermented foods in your diet.

Calorie restriction is only effective when you both *limit calories* and *increase the quality* of what you eat and digest. The fermented foods and liquids you're learning about in this book will allow you to do just this. But they also have a host of other benefits:

— Fermented foods create a healthy inner ecosystem. Fermented foods lay the foundation for our internal garden of microbiota: the "Missing Piece" that must be inside of us, supplying energy for everyday life.

— Fermented foods are a must for immunity. Up to 80 percent of the immune system resides in the gut-associated lymph tissue in our intestines. The microbiota living there play a key role in keeping that region healthy and free of pathogenic (bad) bacteria, and *us* well nourished and immunologically hardy.

— Fermented foods and beverages can be more potent than probiotic supplements. That's because the microbiota obtained from organic foods grown in the ground form powerful synergistic relationships with one another that ensure that they flourish. They must survive in nature, versus being grown in a lab. While probiotic-supplement companies offer ever-increasing numbers of bacteria per capsule, *probiotic foods contain hardier microbiota than those found in these supplements*—and supplements actually work *better* when you have *fermented foods* and *liquids* in your diet.

— Fermented foods provide more nutrients. The microbiota abundant in unpasteurized, fermented foods provide additional enzymes to properly process nutrients, markedly increasing their availability.

— **Fermented foods improve digestion.** The microbiota in fermented foods help protect the gut lining. They also increase the bioavailability of each meal so you can better absorb nutrients, allowing deficiencies to be corrected.

— **Fermented foods are raw . . . but more than raw.** Raw foods may be difficult to digest, especially as we age. Many are very rich in sugars, which make our bodies too acidic, feeding yeast, viruses, and other pathogens. Fermented foods have all the benefits of raw foods . . . including enzymes, antioxidants, and cell messengers such as *polyphenols* and *catechins* . . . yet none of the disadvantages.

— **Fermented foods control cravings.** Carbohydrates, sugar, and alcohol leach minerals from our bones, making our blood more acidic, so avoiding them is essential for restoring our prenatal energy. However, since they are addictive, many people do not have the willpower to resist these cravings. With two related epidemics—obesity and diabetes—threatening to take the lives of many Americans, fermented foods and drinks (such as cultured vegetables and young coconut kefir) become a godsend.

— **Fermented foods allow us to enjoy mildly sweet foods found in nature**. Microbiota eat the sugars in foods and shield us from damage that sugar can often cause. Too much sugar can disrupt the balance of the beneficial flora, but the amount found in natural foods is conducive to their growth. How perfect that we can enjoy the sweet taste of a carrot while our microbiota benefit from the sugar.

— **Fermented foods are detoxifiers.** Due to planetary toxicity, now more than ever we need to put these microbiota to work on cleaning up our environment. Microbes ingest toxins, like pesticides and the mercury found in fish, as well as other harmful materials, and remove them through colonic elimination. (At least 70 percent or more of the weight of the bowel movement is bacteria.)

— **Fermented foods make a healthy "fast food."** These foods and beverages are healthy alternatives to fast food. They are filling, nutrient rich, and easy to digest. Additionally, their high liquid content makes them ideal fast breakfast foods. A smoothie made with fermented milk kefir is a perfect way to start the day for those of us who digest dairy well. A nondairy smoothie made with young coconut kefir is great for those who don't.

— **Fermented foods restore acid/alkaline balance.** Fermented foods are excellent for helping restore the best possible acid/alkaline balance. Because the microbiota are so efficient in promoting colonic absorption of minerals such as calcium and magnesium, our blood can pick up the minerals and carry them out to our cells. With the correct mineral balance, the body remains in a healthy alkaline range. Cancer, diabetes, yeast, and viruses can't grow in an optimal alkaline environment.

— **Fermented foods provide a sour taste for improved digestion.** The sourness of fermented foods (due to the lactic acid produced by the microbiota) stimulates peristaltic movement so that our intestines eliminate properly. To be well balanced, according to Ayurvedic medicine, a great meal should have as many of the six tastes (sweet, sour, salty, bitter, pungent, and astringent) as possible, in the right balance.

Given the healing benefits of fermented foods, it's never too late to start reinforcing your inner ecosystem—and rebuilding your health.

Find the Fermented Foods That Work for You

Fortunately, there are a growing number of options for enjoying fermented foods, and you can choose according to convenience and your own unique palate.

Once again, these are quintessential anti-aging foods. Yes, they are new to many of us and involve a bit of a learning curve, but these fermented foods and drinks are so critical to our vitality and longevity that they are well worth seeking out. In fact, they may be our number one ally in our quest to age "youthfully" and healthfully.

Remember, when fermented, a food or liquid becomes sour. Many of us are not familiar with this taste and only enjoy the sweet and salty tastes. But please eat and drink these sour foods for a week and you'll soon be "hooked." Visit Body Ecology's website (**www .bodyecology.com**) for more articles on fermented foods, and discover how they can help prevent or reverse many health conditions and add many more years to your life.

The following sections feature three especially amazing fermented foods: *cultured vegetables, cultured vegetable juices,* and *young coconut kefir.*

Cultured Vegetables

Cultured or fermented vegetables have been around for thousands of years. Captain Cook took barrels with him on his long voyages to the South Pacific. They protected his crew from developing, and dying from, scurvy.

Indeed, they have been survival foods for many cultures, and we humans might not be here if we hadn't learned how to ferment vegetables as a way to preserve them, providing us with nutrients through long winters. You may be familiar with kimchi, a cultured-vegetable product from Korea consisting of bok choy cabbage, carrots, green onions, ginger, garlic, and hot peppers. And certainly, most of us are familiar with sauerkraut, coined by the Austrians from the German *sauer* (sour) and *Kraut* (greens or plants).

Cultured veggies are raw, cut, and shredded vegetables that have been left to ferment at room temperature. This allows the naturally present lactobacilli and enzymes to proliferate, creating a vitamin-, mineral-, and enzyme-rich superfood.

Keeping in mind that microbes act as alchemists, fermenting vegetables not only increases their nutrient value, but also negates the adverse effects some have on our bodies. For example, cabbage, kale, and collards have a thyroid-suppressing effect when eaten raw—something to be aware of in this day and age when many of us have issues with low thyroid. However, when we ferment them, we still get the benefits of the enzymes found in raw foods, but without the thyroid-suppressing effects.

Certain sweet vegetables—like sweet potatoes and beets—are very rich in sugar; and when they are cooked, they become even sweeter, a problem for many people with conditions such as candida and diabetes. Fermenting allows us to benefit from their nutrients, while the microbiota feed on their natural sugars.

Cultured Vegetable Juices

A small juice glass of cultured veggie juice is perfect with any meal. It provides the sour taste to stimulate digestion, as well as peristalsis to ensure that food moves through your digestive tract with ease. At Body Ecology, we love cultured veggie juice so much that years ago we began to recommend that parents give it to their newborns to help prevent colic, autism, and other disorders that emerge in childhood. A baby may make funny faces at this strange sour taste when given tiny spoonfuls soon after birth, but it helps with digestion of milk and builds a stronger immune system. (*With a strong immune system, a child is less likely to become "infected" by a vaccination and develop autism.*) Another nice plus: When babies are introduced to the sour taste early in life, they don't develop a "sweet tooth." They grow up feeling quite satisfied with the sweetness in a carrot or a berry.

Please share the value of fermented foods and drinks with your children and grandchildren as they see you enjoying small glasses of cultured veggie juice each day.

Recipe for Cultured Veggie Juice

1. Fill a blender with chopped green or red cabbage.
2. Add springwater until blender is ⅔ full.
3. Blend at high speed for 2 minutes.
4. Add package of *L. plantarum* starter culture (easily obtained from **www.bodyecology.com**).
5. Pour mixture into a glass jar with a tight-fitting lid.
6. Let sit at room temperature for 3 days.
7. Strain and place in refrigerator.
8. For a second batch, simply add ½ cup of the first batch to the second instead of the *L. plantarum* starter culture, and it will be ready in 24 hours.

Drink 1½ cups of cultured vegetable juice per day . . . divided throughout the day. We suggest drinking a small juice glass with each meal, as it greatly assists digestion. Consuming several ounces upon waking and at bedtime when the stomach is empty is also wise.

Young Coconut Kefir

Most people are familiar with coconut meat and water from the mature (brown, hairy) coconut. A green coconut is the same food, but younger. The liquid inside is much more like sweet water and is different from prepared coconut milk. Please don't confuse *coconut water* with *coconut milk,* which is actually made from warm water and the meat of the mature coconut. *Coconut water* is the liquid found naturally inside the young coconut. It is full of B vitamins and minerals, especially potassium and sodium—two important minerals for heart and adrenal health. This water has been known for centuries to have a cleansing effect on the liver, kidneys, and heart.

While unfermented coconut water makes a delicious drink on its own, it is too sweet to be *medicinal.* Drinking it will make your body too acidic and encourage the growth of pathogens (viruses and yeast) and tumors. You can still obtain the benefits of this superfood,

however, by *fermenting* the young coconut water, making young coconut kefir—a bubbly, champagne-like drink.

A "Feel-Good" Tonic

Kefir means "feel good" in Turkish. Milk kefir has been called "nature's tranquilizer" or "nature's Prozac" because of its calming effect.
It contains *tryptophan,* an essential amino acid that when combined
with calcium and magnesium helps calm the nervous system. In fact,
the body converts tryptophan into serotonin—a neurotransmitter, or
chemical messenger in the brain allowing for communication between
nerve cells. Serotonin, also referred to as 5-HT, is known to modulate
emotions, mood, memory and learning, temperature regulation, behavior, cardiovascular function, muscle contraction, endocrine regulation,
sleep, and appetite. This makes it especially helpful for people who are
depressed, high-strung, or nervous; or who have trouble sleeping (serotonin converts to the sleep hormone melatonin)—not to mention for
those wishing to improve memory function, especially as they age. Kefir
is very easy to make at home with Body Ecology's Kefir Starter.

Today it is much easier to obtain fresh coconut water for fermenting than it once was. Thai coconuts have the sweetest water
in the world, which is best for fermenting. Exotic Superfoods now
imports fresh, frozen *organic* coconut water from Thailand. Many
Whole Foods Markets and other health-food stores are carrying it in
their frozen-food section. Not only is coconut water in cans or aseptic
packages pasteurized, but it isn't sweet enough to ferment. CocoKefir
and inner-ēco are two companies that now manufacture young coconut kefir. You can find this amazing healing probiotic in your local
health-food store.

From the Physician's Desk

"We have at least 10 trillion cells in our
bodies and 100 trillion microbes in the form
of bacteria, parasites, and fungi. Managing
these microbes should be a top priority."

One hundred years ago, people such as Nobel Prize winner Dr. Élie Metchnikov talked and wrote about the anti-aging benefits of fermented foods. Fortunately, we are once again beginning to realize the importance of this overlooked area of health. However, there are parts of the world that have always routinely used fermented foods. When I was traveling with my wife in Denmark and Sweden, there would be jars of fermented yogurt on the table to take with meals. It was simply a natural part of the diet. In fact, fermented foods have been used for thousands of years in many regions of the world, ranging from Europe, Africa, and the Middle East to India, China, and Japan, where they depended upon bacterial cultures long before refrigeration was available.

Certainly, refrigeration has been a wonderful addition to life—and has saved a lot of lives—but we've also lost something vital in the process by forgetting about the value of culturing foods. Once again, we are now revisiting this most valuable technology as a cornerstone of health.

There is another major reason why cultured foods should be a part of every meal. Every year 70 million people in the United States check into the ER due to food poisoning, regardless of whether they eat at home or in restaurants. This problem can be diminished with the regular intake of fermented foods, or *probiotics*. Science has shown that fermented vegetables and drinks fill the gut with beneficial bacteria. These probiotic-laden foods make their own biofilms and antibiotics *(bacteriocins)*, which kill, disable, and crowd out pathogenic bacteria.

Beneficial microbiota are basically an excellent insurance policy. In healthy people, the percentage of pathogenic bacteria in the body is much lower than the amounts of neutral and beneficial bacteria. When we become sick or get out of balance in some way, then the pathogenic bacteria can start multiplying, and literally take on a life of their own. Unless we are proactive, these pathogens disrupt the microbial balance, leading to often-permanent degenerative diseases.

Remember, we have at least 10 trillion cells in our bodies and 100 trillion microbes—mostly bacteria, with some fungi, parasites, and viruses. The necessity of managing these microbes to the degree we can should be obvious. Yet most of us have little or no notion of friendly bacteria or how to culture our foods.

I believe that if you were going to make only one beneficial change in your lifestyle and health in the next year, it should be to begin integrating fermented foods into your diet. Most health programs talk about the importance of healthy carbs, exercise, getting your omega-3s, and so forth. The Body Ecology program, however, is one of the few to address the importance of the inner ecosystem and bacteria management through fermented foods.

— *Leonard Smith, M.D.*

CHAPTER 7

SUGAR:
How Sweet It Isn't

For decades enlightened health professionals were implicating sugar as a dangerous poison and major culprit in aging. How can we satisfy our taste for sugar without harming ourselves?

During World War II, sugar and sweetened dairy products such as ice cream were rationed. Indeed, they were thought to be luxury items. Once the war ended, the restriction was lifted, and sugar consumption increased dramatically. Suddenly, highly sweetened foods—including refined, puffy, sweetened cereals and a number of brands of soda pop—began hitting America's supermarket shelves. The switch from farm-grown foods to processed ones, where sugar was often used as a preservative and "flavor enhancer," further shoved consumers down the high-sugar path, and coincided with a continual decline in our health.

Today it is well accepted that when we eat *dietary* sugar, it causes a yo-yo effect on our *blood* sugar. Dietary sugar creates a temporary *spike* in our glucose, followed by a dramatic *drop* in glucose, causing our energy to plummet. To regain energy, we crave and then eat another sweet-tasting food or drink that will send it soaring once again.

Most of us have been addicted to sugar since infancy, and now as we age, we are once again experiencing multiple *epidemics* of poor health, including obesity, diabetes, Alzheimer's, cancer, and digestive diseases such as Crohn's. Obviously, to reverse the aging process, we must stop the madness and avoid the consumption of sugars. We must do so for our own well-being, but especially for the well-being of our children and grandchildren, because autism, obesity, diabetes, and cancer have now become *their* epidemics.

When you think about how much sugar is found in processed foods today, it's pretty scary. Statistics say that more than 20 percent of the total calories we consume each day are from refined sugars. Sugar is hidden in our foods under the guise of *sucrose, dextrose, maltose, sorbitol, turbinado*—and more. In fact, each year the average person consumes his or her body weight in these empty, dangerous calories—plus more than 20 pounds of corn syrup.

Death by Spoonful

Sugar may "help the medicine go down," but it also depletes us of our prenatal life force, our *jing*. And, unfortunately, death by sugar is usually slow and can be *physically* painful. As my friend Dr. Joe Mercola stated on his popular health website (**www.mercola.com**): "The health dangers ingested sugar creates when habitually imposed upon human physiology are certain. Simple sugars have been observed to aggravate asthma, muster mental illness, move mood swings, provoke personality changes, nourish nervous disorders, hurry heart disease, deliver diabetes, grow gallstones, hasten hypertension, add arthritis, and on top of all of that . . . it will kill you!"[1]

If Joe's words of warning that sugar is slowly but surely killing us may seem a bit too dramatic to you, there is much research to support his statements. Recent cell-metabolism experiments suggest that when worms were fed glucose as part of their diets, they lived for a *shorter* amount of time than those that *never consumed* it, according to researchers from the University of Jena, Germany.[2] If these findings in worms hold for humans, then even in healthy people, the breakdown of sugar into glucose has detrimental effects on life span.

Sugar consumption may not only shorten our lives, it may make the quality of our final years quite a bit bleaker as well. A study conducted by the American Society for Biochemistry and Molecular Biology showed that high sugar consumption in an otherwise-normal diet could affect the progression of Alzheimer's disease. Using a genetic mouse model, researchers found that mice that were given 10 percent sugar water showed poorer learning and memory retention than the control group, and their brains contained more than twice as many amyloid plaque deposits, which play a major role in the destruction of nerve cells and are an anatomical hallmark of Alzheimer's.[3] The connection between diabetes and Alzheimer's has long been known. In fact, some scientists even refer to Alzheimer's as "type 3 diabetes."

And Sugar Makes You Look and Feel Really Old, Too

Dietary-sugar molecules bond to protein molecules and create "cross-linked proteins," meaning that proteins start bonding to each other. This is called *glycosylation* (see Chapter 2 and the glycation theory of aging). Basically, tissues stiffen and do not function efficiently. Cataracts are an example of stiffening of our eye lenses, and we lose our sight. Stiffening skin tissue becomes tough, yellow, and leathery. You can imagine what it looks like to see the results of cross-linked proteins accumulating in cartilage, lung tissue, arteries, and tendons.

Sugar hardens, weakens, and poisons every system in the body, including the endocrine system. As hormone production slowly fades away—especially in our adrenals and the pituitary, which produces growth hormone—our sex drive diminishes, men become impotent, and energy wanes, causing us to lose our ability to cleanse out toxins. We become more and more constipated, and our intestines fill with decaying fecal material. Signs that we are poisoning ourselves are gray hair, weak fingernails, bone loss, and sarcopenia (loss of lean muscle, replaced by fat). Perhaps worst of all is that our brains literally shrink and develop holes.

Because sugar is devoid of vitamins, minerals, and fiber, it creates an acidic body—and one day, a checkup at the doctor's office reveals that we have cancer cells growing rapidly out of control. *As powerful as any drug, sugar lifts us up, only to knock us right back down.* It has long been known that sugar's addictive properties and withdrawal symptoms are similar to narcotics. Are we shocked, then, that most of us are sugar addicts?

Artificial Sweeteners . . . On Their Way Out!

While it may have seemed smart at one point to turn to artificial sweeteners such as aspartame (NutraSweet and Equal) and sucralose (Splenda), we now know that these alternatives are a double-edged sword. The average American consumes more than 50 pounds of artificial sweetener per year, often unwittingly, in snacks and soda pop. Aspartame has been found to create side effects such as memory loss, blurry vision, and headaches.

Even if you were to risk these side effects in exchange for weight loss, evidence is now showing that aspartame actually contributes to obesity. One of its ingredients, the amino acid *phenylalanine,* blocks serotonin, which plays a role in controlling cravings. The effect on your body may be that you start to crave all of those high-carbohydrate, processed foods that can sabotage your dieting goals.

Sucralose has elicited similar findings, such as enlargement of the liver and kidneys, shrinking of the thymus gland (which plays a role in immunity and disease fighting), lymph atrophy, decreased red-blood-cell count, decreased fetal body weight, and diarrhea, just to name a few.

Stevia has none of these side effects, and is all natural! It has no calories, is low on the glycemic index, and produces no increase in blood-sugar levels.

It should come as no surprise that our children and grandchildren face an even grimmer future. A recent study by researchers at the Royal Veterinary College in London found that mothers who eat junk food during pregnancy and while breast-feeding may be putting their children at risk for overeating and developing obesity. The study was carried out on an animal model, in which researchers observed rats fed a diet of processed junk food during pregnancy and lactation. The rats gave birth to offspring that overate and showed a preference for foods rich in fat, sugar, and salt, compared to the offspring of rat mothers given regular feed. *The implications for humans are obvious.*[4]

In our grandchildren, we can clearly see the effects of generations of sugar consumption: early puberty, anxiety, depression, weight gain, confused minds, drug and alcohol addiction, and, sadly, increasing juvenile criminal behavior.

But statistics also show that many of us have become very concerned about the amount of sugar in our diets today. We are taking greater responsibility for our own health and for that of our children and grandchildren. We are reading labels more. We want a change.

Sugar and the Principle of Balance

At Body Ecology, we are committed to helping you reduce your sugar consumption dramatically, and the Body Ecology way of eating is almost totally free of sugars. Yet, we also recognize the need that we humans have for the sweet taste. Remember that according to Ayurvedic medicine, we humans desire and even need six tastes: sweet, salty, sour, bitter, pungent, and astringent. In a well-prepared meal, the Ayurvedic cook balances the sweet taste with the other tastes on the plate. With this balance, we feel satisfied, and our organs will be receiving what they need. In other words, the sweet taste is just as important as salty, bitter, sour, and so on, so we should not feel guilty when we desire it. It has a clear purpose along with all the other tastes and senses.

All foods have a positive and negative—a front and a back. In small amounts, sugar increases energy, especially in demanding situations such as physical labor or exercise. It also nourishes our sense organs and promotes strength. But it is well understood that sugar "increases tissue," meaning it causes us to become larger, even obese. In addition, the character of this taste is cold, damp, and heavy on digestion. When there's too much, we create an imbalance, experiencing lethargy, mucous conditions, constipation, and a general heaviness.

Overcoming Our Cravings for and Addiction to Sugar

The first step in overcoming a serious sugar addiction is to quell our desire for it. The sour taste does just that. We can be satisfied by eating or drinking sour, fermented foods, as discussed at length in the previous chapter.

Once you add fermented foods and beverages to your diet, you will begin to lose much of your desire for sweet foods. In fact, you will start to really be able to taste the natural sweetness in fruits and sweet vegetables and be perfectly satisfied with these. Candy bars, pastries, and colas will become overly sweet.

Have you ever noticed how, soon after a sugar binge, out of the blue you crave salty foods such as chips? Or you might suddenly begin to crave an animal-protein meal? These cravings are your body's way of trying to maintain balance. Sea salt, an alkaline food, provides valuable minerals that are lost when acidic, mineral-leaching sugars are consumed. Animal proteins also contain salt and minerals in the blood.

Adrenal fatigue becomes the norm as we age, so to get a boost of temporary energy, many of us reach for sugar and/or salty foods. We seesaw back and forth, wanting both, but those sugary snacks that give us a short-lived boost of energy drain the adrenals even further, and a vicious cycle results. Fermented foods, on the other hand, help nourish the body so efficiently that our blood sugar stays stable, minerals are extracted and retained to build our adrenals, and cravings disappear.

Dehydration

A major cause of cravings for sweets is that your body needs water. Before you succumb to a sugar craving, try this: Sit down for five or ten minutes and drink two glasses of mineral-rich water. You'll be amazed by how well this works. You can also add stevia and lemon juice to your water to satisfy your sweet tooth. Even better, add a few ounces of a probiotic liquid such as young coconut kefir or Body Ecology's CocoBiotic.

Sugar and the Principle of Acid and Alkaline

As you know, when there is too much sugar in your body, an overly acidic condition results. An acidic body provides an ideal haven for pathogens such as viruses, fungi, and cancer cells. Viruses, for example, have been shown to create serious chronic inflammation, which is a major cause of aging. They have been linked to heart disease as well.

Sugar and the Principle of Food Combining

Sugar should always be eaten alone. When you combine it with another food, it creates gas.

Sweets, the Body Ecology Way

There are several natural ways to sweeten your foods and beverages that are healthy for your body. You may not have heard of all of them because they don't have billion-dollar marketing budgets behind them, but they are quietly entering health-food stores or are sold on the Internet.

Stevia

An extraordinarily sweet herb, stevia is 200 to 300 times sweeter than sugar—and yet, it's nearly calorie free! Stevia is a member of the chrysanthemum family (closely related to chamomile and tarragon) and is totally safe.

Stevia is available as crushed green leaves; as a crude, greenish-brown syrup; as a white powder extract; and as an easy-to-use liquid concentrate prepared from the white powder extract. In its crude, unprocessed form, the stevia plant has been consumed for centuries by the Indians of South America. The Japanese, looking for a safe sweetener substitute, developed the process used to extract two primary compounds, *rebaudioside* and *stevioside,* from the plant to create a delicious white powder. Stevia has now been enjoyed and used safely in Japan for the past 30-plus years.

The crude green stevia leaves and syrup have a strong licorice-like flavor that many do not like. So while they do have medicinal value (such as helping to heal wounds and preventing dental cavities), they are not recommended as a sweetener. The white powder doesn't have this aftertaste if used sparingly.

Neither the whole plant nor the extract will raise blood sugar, making it safe for diabetics. An excellent flavor enhancer when used in very small amounts, stevia is especially tasty in dairy and with fruits.

Stevia has been tested in human and animal studies in many major countries, including Japan, Brazil, and Israel, with no negative side effects. Ironically, of the more than 9,000 complaints filed with the FDA since 1985, about 80 percent are related to NutraSweet, yet *it* is still on the market.[5] Once the patent on aspartame had expired, more and more natural alternative sweeteners began to appear on the market. Not all are safe, however. Aspartame, Acesulfame K, and Splenda are not part of the Body Ecology program.

The Story of Stevia

Years ago, I was instrumental in bringing stevia to the United States and published a book called *Stevia: Nature's Calorie-Free Sweetener.* The story behind this is that stevia was a huge threat to the food conglomerate Monsanto, when they still had the patent for aspartame (sold under the labels of Equal and NutraSweet). Someone (no one knew for sure who) petitioned the FDA to raid those tea companies that were using the green stevia leaves in their tea bags. Stevia was then banned from being imported in the U.S.

I led a grassroots movement; and soon, with the help of Drs. Robert Atkins, Andrew Weil, and Julian Whitaker, tens of thousands of people were safely using and enjoying the white powder extract. What an interesting twist of fate that Coca-Cola, Pepsi, and Cargill, which now want to use stevia extract in their beverages, have recently obtained approval from the FDA! Personally, I see this as a victory for all of us who fought to bring stevia into the U.S.

When purchasing stevia, be aware that there are different strengths available, some of which you may like less than others. At Body Ecology, we prefer a stevia *liquid concentrate* for its convenience. The liquid form is great for those who are just starting to experiment with stevia, because you can easily control the amount you add to beverages and foods. The white powder can be more difficult to work with, resulting in oversweetening your food. Many people tell us that our own delicious stevia concentrate is the best-tasting product on the market. It is available at: **www.bodyecology.com.**

Lakanto

Lakanto has been in use in Japan since 1996 and is served in thousands of restaurants and hospitals. It is recommended (not just approved) by the Japanese minister of health as a food for special dietary uses, and it has GRAS (Generally Recognized As Safe) approval in the United States.

What is great about Lakanto is its absolutely delicious taste, and unlike stevia, you can bake with it. You use it just like you would sugar and can even sprinkle it on your food. (Stevia is too strong to "sprinkle." In fact, a tiny bit can be too much, and you will ruin the taste of your food or drink.)

Lakanto is made from a unique patented combination of erythritol and a pure extract of luo han guo, an exotic vine fruit cultivated mainly in East Asia. Erythritol is unlike any other sugar alcohol because it is made from the process of fermentation. The sugar in corn is fermented, so those sensitive to corn can tolerate Lakanto quite well. All other sugar alcohols (maltitol, sorbitol, and xylitol) are made by hydrogenation. This may explain why Lakanto does not cause the symptoms of diarrhea that some people experience when they eat a food or chew gum made with the other sugar alcohols. Luo han guo has been used in traditional Chinese medicine since ancient times to treat a variety of ailments, such as chronic cough, heat stroke, larynx infections, and constipation.

Lakanto is an excellent choice for people who want to combat age, who want to lose weight, or who are insulin resistant or diabetic. It registers "0" on the glycemic index and causes no rise in serum insulin or blood-sugar levels. It tastes similar to maple sugar or toffee, and because it is not altered by heat, it is excellent for baking and cooking. A recipe book is available online at **www.bodyecology.com**.

Xylitol and Erythritol

Xylitol and erythritol are both called "sugar alcohols." And what is a sugar alcohol?

There are two kinds of carbohydrates: (1) *available* carbohydrates, those that the body can use and metabolize; and (2) *unavailable,* also known as "non-glycemic," meaning they have no calories. These zero-calorie, non-glycemic carbs are not used as energy by the body and therefore do not raise blood-sugar levels. This means they will not conflict with your low-carb diet and will not spike blood glucose. A healthy, natural sweetener, xylitol is considered to be an "unavailable" carbohydrate sweetener and is extracted from fruits, vegetables, and birch cellulose.

Xylitol is clinically proven to fight and lessen the occurrence of inner-ear infection. It also has many benefits for teeth, making it a natural replacement for fluoride. These proven benefits include: reducing plaque, fighting cavities, reducing the secretion of plaque acids, and facilitating the re-mineralization of tooth enamel. Additionally, xylitol may help protect against group B strep and has been given to mothers in prenatal clinics.

Erythritol has these wonderful properties as well.

Xylitol and erythritol are low on the glycemic index, and like stevia, are safe for diabetics and hypoglycemics. They look and taste similar to sugar, with 40 percent fewer calories. You can purchase xylitol and erythritol in your health-food store. Some people are sensitive to xylitol, and excessive amounts may cause digestive issues, including diarrhea. Erythritol is made from a different process using fermentation and rarely has negative side effects.

Eliminating sugar from your diet may be the most important first step you take in impeding the aging process. It can be challenging, but by including fermented foods and beverages in your diet, you can manage and eventually get over the desire for sweets.

Sugar is not the only area of our diet where we have been perilously "duped." As you will see in the next chapter, we have also been misled about the importance of healthy fats and oils in a well-rounded diet.

CHAPTER 8

FATS:
The Good, the Bad, and the Ones That Make Us Ugly

Demonized, traditional fats and unrefined extra-virgin oils are your secret weapon against many of the common diseases of aging, such as osteoporosis, macular degeneration, hormone decline, and dementia.

When it comes to progress, not all change is good. Many of the innovations of the 20th century that brought us convenience have cost us something in return. The lightbulb and computer have had both a positive and a negative impact on human health. We can add the modern-day supermarket to the list.

In 1930, Michael Cullen opened the first supermarket in Queens, New York. This seemingly progressive action would have a profoundly *negative* influence on the *quality* of foods eaten around the world.

Supermarkets liberated mothers from the kitchen because they had to make fewer trips to the store and spent less time shopping. But, because convenience became most important in the mind of the American consumer, other issues began to emerge. Products needed to stay on shelves for longer periods of time, and "just-picked freshness" was becoming less of a priority. Shelf stability was a problem for fats and oils because fatty acids, when exposed to heat, light, and oxygen, become damaged. The oils that contain these fatty acids turn rancid and poisonous to eat. Freshly pressed or *unrefined oils* with fragile fatty acids were not ideal for traveling great distances—or for sitting on supermarket shelves for lengthy periods of time. To solve this problem, "food scientists" and manufacturers of vegetable oils extended shelf life by changing or removing all of the *beneficial* fatty acids.

We were a trusting nation then. Parents had confidence in the newly emerging miracles of modern nutritional science . . . man could improve upon nature. "Better" fats, like Crisco, became the new staple—after all . . . "Cooks who know trust Crisco." Believing in what they saw in those ads, few questioned if it was wise or healthy to eat these "plastic," nutritionally useless oils. But alas, to make foods "shelf stable," we altered and desecrated them, thumbing our noses at the "real foods" that had fueled our bodies for thousands of years. You might say we sold our bodies and souls for shelf life.

Now, 50 years later, the consequences of processing and depleting the nutrients in almost every food and drink that passes our lips, *especially altering our fats and oils,* have shaped and will continue to shape the outcome of our health for generations to come.

The Toll That Keeps on Taking

In our younger years, we could eat greasy French fries and pizza and be relatively immune to their effects, but the toll of eating these bad fats and oils has been accumulating year after year. Our prenatal jing has been depleted through decades of bad choices.

The good news is that, while bad fats are still all around us in many of our favorite foods, for the first time we also have a superior collection of very fine fats and oils to include in our rejuvenation arsenal.

The science behind fats and oils is more complex than most of us want or need to know. Here's the solution in a nutshell: *Avoid bad fats as if the quality of your life depended on it (because it does), and eat the good fats that your own unique body thrives on.*

This chapter will spell out the basics: why to eat fats, choosing the right ones, and learning how to use the good ones to prevent diseases of aging.

Big, Bad Saturated Fats: The Lie Lives On . . .

From the moment we were conceived, saturated fats were an important part of our prenatal diet. In the womb, saturated fat played a vital role in our brain and bone development. Later healthy human milk supplied us with the saturated fat needed for our high-energy requirements and rapidly growing bodies.

Clearly, if saturated fat is indispensable to our early infant survival, does it make sense to eliminate it from our diet now? Is the abandonment of this brain-nourishing fat and the adoption of *margarine* one of the reasons why dementia and Alzheimer's have become so prevalent?

What about our aging bones—and osteopenia and osteoporosis? Milk fat helps "drive" the minerals in milk (calcium and phosphorus) into our bones. While more than 40 percent of our bone mass is achieved between the ages of 12 and 18, we must consciously be mindful of adding minerals into our "bone bank account" throughout our lives. Saturated fat, especially from ghee and raw butter, helps us assimilate those minerals.

We Never Lose Our Need for Saturated Fat

With breast milk no longer an option for us, the adult version of saturated fat can be obtained from eating butter and ghee. And the other important fats in breast milk, which provide us with DHA and EPA fatty acids, can be found in fish oil.

Ideally, butter should be eaten raw. Ghee, also called clarified butter, is ideal for cooking. (In India, it is a tradition to place a spoonful of ghee on a baby's tongue at birth. The Tibetan monks drink as many as five cups of ghee each day for energy and warmth.) If you find that you thrive on *fermented milk products* in the form of kefir, yogurt, or raw cheeses, you can obtain saturated milk fat in these foods as well. Although our saturated-fat needs may not be as great as an infant's, adult brains and bones can benefit immeasurably from some saturated milk fat.

Blaming Saturated Fats for Heart Disease

This may surprise you, but in the early 1900s, we were a nation that ate mostly saturated fats from butter, lard (rendered fat from pork), tallow (rendered fat from beef or mutton), palm oil, and coconut oil. We only ate a very small amount of olive oil. *Heart disease was rare.* But then we decided to "fool Mother Nature."

In 1902, German chemist Wilhelm Normann patented the process to make hydrogenated vegetable oils. By 1911, Procter & Gamble had bought the rights and made Crisco commercially available for frying and baking.[1]

By 1950, heart disease had become a leading cause of death in the U.S. Research indicated that *vegetable* oils were linked to this increase. But in 1960 the American Heart Association (AHA) issued a statement indicating that *saturated* fat correlated with heart disease. For obvious reasons, the vegetable-oil industry—corn, soybean, and peanut—began to attack *saturated* fats, blaming meats, eggs, cheese, butter, and tropical oils (palm and coconut) as the heart-disease culprits. Almost five decades later, with our more sophisticated understanding of fats, the *most up-to-date research indicates that small amounts of healthy saturated fats help in preventing heart disease.*

But from 1960 on, we Americans began eating a "low-fat diet" that included more *refined, hydrogenated* vegetable-based fats such as margarine made from corn, soybean, and safflower oils. This was a tragic mistake that has contributed to epidemics of obesity, eating disorders, hormone imbalances, infertility, brain disorders such as Alzheimer's, ADHD, and depression; as well as cancers, diabetes, and, ironically, *an increase in heart disease.*

The Science of Fats

There are two types of fat (or lipids) found circulating in our bloodstream: *cholesterol* and *triglycerides.* Both of these are necessary for life. Cholesterol acts as a precursor for our sexual hormones such as estrogen and testosterone and even vitamin D (really a hormone). It is an essential part of the membrane of a cell. Triglycerides are important in the production of energy for most cells in the body (but not brain cells). They are stored in the body's fat cells until needed for energy.

In spite of these benefits, elevated triglycerides have been linked to obesity, heart disease, diabetes, and surprisingly, even depression. *You can be on a low-fat diet and still have elevated triglycerides in your bloodstream. Why? Because inactivity, drinking alcohol, and taking drugs (including birth-control pills, steroids, and diuretics) can raise triglyceride levels. An underactive thyroid can also put you at risk. But perhaps the biggest cause of elevated triglycerides is that we eat so many sugar- and carb-laden foods today.*

When saturated fats and extra-virgin oils—all very flavorful—were eliminated, foods became tasteless. No one would buy them, so our "food scientists" solved this problem by increasing the amount of sugar in them. When we have a diet high in sugars (bread, pasta, cereals, doughnuts, sodas, white rice, and the like), the liver produces more triglycerides than we need. In other words, when *sugars* are not burned immediately as energy, they create elevated triglycerides that lead to heart disease, diabetes, and certainly obesity . . . even in our children.

The Creation of the Molecular Misfits

Once traditional fats were vilified, food manufacturers saw a perfect opportunity to gain control of the market. The process of *hydrogenation* allowed oils such as refined soybean, corn, and canola oil . . . normally in a liquid form . . . to be changed into a *solid* form to create margarines, spreads, and shortenings. The result were trans-fatty acids—known as "molecular misfits." Trans fats lower good cholesterol (HDL) and impair blood-vessel function.

For years trans-fatty acids showed up in commercially made shortenings, margarines, and fats usually called "hydrogenated vegetable oils" and "partially hydrogenated vegetable oils." Even after the health risks associated with consuming trans-fatty acids became highly publicized several years ago, we still find them in French fries, chicken nuggets, breakfast cereals, crackers, doughnuts, candies, Girl Scout cookies, and every kid's favorite, macaroni and "cheese." You are eating them when you ask for "butter" at your local movie theater.

Although we have known for some time that trans fats are poisonous, members of the edible-oil industry do not want them identified. Finally, however, new labeling laws are changing this. In 2005, New York City officials announced that all 20,000 restaurants must remove trans fats from their menu. In January 2010 California became the first *state* to ban them. Major chains such as Kentucky Fried Chicken, Wendy's, and McDonald's have caved under the pressure and have stopped cooking with them. But in many cases restaurants are still using trans fats in their cooking oils, arguing that trans-fat-free oils will adversely change the taste of foods and along with it, their sales.[2] You should be aware of this when choosing to dine out.

Speaking of Which . . . Don't Forget about Fried Foods

Fried foods also contribute to the diseases of aging. When oils are heated to high temperatures—as in frying, roasting, and baking—toxic molecules are formed. *HNE,* a highly toxic compound, accumulates each time polyunsaturated vegetable oil is reheated and reused for frying.

Acrylamide is a chemical formed when carbohydrates and starchy foods are baked, roasted, fried, or grilled—think French fries, potato chips, cookies, and bread. At high temperatures (338 degrees Fahrenheit/170 degrees Celsius), the sugar in these foods reacts with a protein and forms this neurotoxin—which has been linked to reproductive issues. For these reasons, staying away from fried foods is part of the Body Ecology Way of Life.

Be Suspicious of What You Find in Many Popular Health-Food Stores

Watch out for the oils that are simply marked "cold-pressed" or "expeller-pressed." Even if they are found in health-food stores, they do not have the same benefits as *unrefined* oils. A lot of what are being marketed as "healthy" oils, such as *refined* canola oil, lack color and flavor and are deficient in nutrients and fatty acids. Our livers are simply not designed to handle them. With the goal of extending shelf life, all of the beneficial fatty acids have been removed from these "plastic" oils, making them nutritionally useless.

We've been eating *refined* oils for more than five generations here in the U.S., a legacy that now affects all generations currently living and those who are yet to be born. A more sophisticated understanding of the science behind fats and oils clearly shows that bad fats communicate bad information to the body. While *good fats can silence genes* that might be expressed as heart disease, Alzheimer's, and diabetes, *bad ones express or turn these genes on.*

So, now that we've learned a little of the history of America's "low-fat controversy," let's move on to the benefits of healthy fats and oils, and what foods we need to eat to obtain them.

Let's Simplify— the Good Things Good Fat Can Do

In a nutshell, we eat fats and oils to obtain their essential fatty acids and their other important fat-soluble nutrients, including the vitamins A, D, E, and K. Fatty acids are the key components of fats. Fats provide energy and satiety, regulate cholesterol, create a stronger immune system, and relieve pain and arthritis. They are needed for health and certainly play a major role in how we age—or don't.

Healthy, unrefined oils are being used in alternative medical clinics and spas around the world to fight depression, emotional disorders, ADHD, autism, and even schizophrenia. When eaten in their extra-virgin, unrefined state, fats and oils are also quite delicious, so they provide us with pleasure and enjoyment as well.

Here are just a few of the many anti-aging benefits of fats.

Beauty

Fats make us look great! They moisturize and replenish our skin, and they keep our hormone levels from declining, a main reason we begin to lose some of our youthful "sexiness." The right fats can cool down inflammation in the body, a significant factor in aging.

Vision

Fats are essential to the eye's rods and cones and are critical to many metabolic functions inside the eye. Some experts believe healthy fats in foods such as nuts may have the same positive effect on our eyes as they do on our hearts. The healthy fats in nuts may prevent total fat from clogging the "arteries" of our eyes. Given that macular degeneration and other diseases of the eyes, such as cataracts, are related to inflammation, a diet rich in leafy-green vegetables and omega-3 fatty foods that protect the body from free-radical damage is essential.

Brain Function

Fats make up 60 percent of the brain and are essential to brain function, including learning abilities, memory retention, and emotional equilibrium.

Bone Density

Osteoporosis affects more than 25 million Americans a year, mostly women. Although there is certainly a genetic predisposition (women whose mothers had osteoporosis are more likely to have it), heredity does not mean osteoporosis is a foregone conclusion. There is a clear link between a healthy diet and exercise and lowered susceptibility to osteoporosis. A diet high in a variety of healthy fats affects overall mineral density and absorption in the bones, helps the body properly utilize bone-related vitamins such as vitamin D, and reduces the chance of bone loss. In fact, certain fats (raw butter, ghee, fish oil, and the fat in egg yolk) actually contain vitamin D.

The Endocrine System—Hormone Production

Fats help regulate hormones, and by the time we reach our mid-40s, hormone issues become a greater concern. If your diet is deficient in good-quality fats, it is also likely that your body is not producing hormones in adequate amounts. Fats are required to make hormones and hormone-like substances called *prostaglandins* found in every tissue, cell, and organ in the body. By contrast, unhealthy fats and trans fats actually interfere with healthy hormone production by blocking the pathways in your body that produce hormones.

Where to Find Fats

If you have even the slightest interest in nutrition, you are probably well aware that fats are broken down into different groupings—*saturated, polyunsaturated, monounsaturated,* and *trans fats.* Here is a list of the fats in each category; **those recommended by Body Ecology are in boldface.** Remember: purchase these only if they are labeled as *unrefined, virgin,* or *raw.*

Saturated Fatty Acids

- **Butter, ghee,** and **egg yolk**
- Lard from pigs; tallow and suet from cattle, sheep, and lamb
- Whole-fat milk, cream, and cheese
- Meats and meat products such as sausage; poultry such as chicken, goose, and duck
- Plant sources such as **avocado, palm oil, coconut oil, coconut milk,** and **coconut meat**

Raw butter is delicious melted on your vegetables and grain-like seeds; ghee, red-palm oil, and coconut oil are great for cooking. All four can also be taken by the spoonful as a fatty-acid supplement. Once you correct any nutritional deficiencies, you will need a lesser amount of these in your diet on a daily basis. The cholesterol in egg yolk is an important fat for both growing and aging brains.

Polyunsaturated Fatty Acids

- **Nuts and their oils**—macadamia, walnut, pecan, pine nut, and almond

- **Seeds and their oils**—flax, hemp, pumpkin, canola (note that unrefined canola has an unpleasant aftertaste), chia, tea, sacha inchi, and sesame

- **Oily fish**—salmon, fish eggs, cod-liver oil, and a variety of small fish, such as anchovies and sardines

- Vegetables—corn oil (not recommended)

- Legumes—peanut and soybean oil (not recommended)

Time for an Oil Change!

Looking for a super-nutritious cooking oil? Try this Body Ecology blend:

1 cup ghee
1 cup coconut oil
3 Tbsp. red-palm oil

While still in their original glass jars, set oils down into very warm water to melt them. Mix together in a clean glass jar. This multipurpose cooking oil is great for sautéing. You can also take a spoonful each day as a supplement.

Other great oils you may not have considered:

- **Ghee**—less mucus-forming than butter; contains butyric and caprylic acid; has antimicrobial properties; absorbs directly, for quick energy

- **Coconut oil**—excellent for thyroid; easily digested; has anti-fungal, antiviral properties
- **Pumpkin-seed oil**—nourishes the ovaries, bladder, and digestive tract; helps fight parasites and is a source of zinc, iron, and niacin
- **Red-palm oil**—contains vitamins A and E and lauric acid; has antifungal, antiviral properties
- **Borage-seed oil**—helps regulate a woman's hormones
- **Evening-primrose oil**—helps regulate hormones (Barlean's Essential Woman is a blend of evening-primrose and flax oil: **www.barleans.com**)
- **Flaxseed oil**—a vegetarian source of omega-3s
- **Cod-liver oil**—great to take in colder months for omega-3s and vitamins A and D
- **Avocado oil** (unrefined)
- **Walnut oil** (available from **www.florahealth.com** and **www.lanogalerawalnutoil.com**)
- **Salmon oil**—rich in omega-3s; great for weight control (available from **www.vitalchoice.com**)
- **Marine-lipid oils**—includes anchovy, sardine, and krill oil
- **Green-lipped-mussel oil** from New Zealand
- **Hemp-seed oil**—contains a good ratio of omega-3 and omega-6 (available from **www.manitobaharvest.com**)
- **Raw butter**—contains lipase, which helps digest fat; and butyric acid, for healthier intestinal microbiota

There are also some flavorful oil blends:

- **Omega Nutrition** produces a blend called Essential Balance Junior—a mixture of flax oil, extra-virgin olive oil, and pumpkin-seed oil, plus flax particulate and natural butterscotch flavor. Their Garlic Chili Flax Seed Oil is also delicious (**www.omeganutrition.com**).
- **Foods Alive** produces flax oil blended with organic garlic and paprika (**www.foodsalive.com**).
- **Green Pasture** produces cinnamon-flavored cod-liver oil (**www.greenpasture.org**).
- **Barlean's** makes a wildly popular line of "swirl" oils (**www.barleans.com**). They are excellent by the spoonful for children of all ages and are also loved by adults. Use them in your green morning-smoothie recipes.

Vegetable and legume oils such as corn, soybean, and peanut oil must be strictly avoided if you want to stay young. They have been refined and stripped of any valuable fatty acids. They have also been bleached and deodorized. To your liver and gallbladder, they read like plastic. To rejuvenate, you must give these organs your special attention, and a good first step would be to stop poisoning them!

The rest of the oils mentioned can be obtained in their extra-virgin, unrefined state. They can be drizzled on your vegetables and grain-like seeds. They can also be taken by the spoonful as a fatty-acid supplement.

Monunsaturated Fatty Acids

- Fruits such as **olives** and **olive oil**, **avocados** and **avocado oil**, and **tea-seed oil** (not to be confused with tea-*tree* oil)

If you are wondering exactly how *much* fat is recommended, remember that your body is unique. As there are a number of aspects to consider, I cannot suggest, as most diet books do, to eat a certain percentage of saturated fats or to avoid them completely. You must decide this for yourself.

Whatever you decide, if you follow the Body Ecology Way of Life, you can enjoy eating a delicious *variety* of all the recommended *organic, unrefined fats and oils* throughout the week. Slowly but surely you'll watch your youthful vitality return.

Choosing the Right Fats and Oils

As previously mentioned, it's critical to only purchase oils that are *organic* and *unrefined* for the best health benefits. But it's also important to choose a *variety* of oils, so you get the full range of essential fatty acids.

While there are hundreds of fatty acids found in nature, two unsaturated fatty acids, *omega-3* and *omega-6,* are called essential fatty acids (EFAs), because it is *essential* that we obtain these from fats in our food. If the body has these two, it can manufacture the other important fatty acids it needs.

Most of us get ample amounts of omega-6. It is the omega-3s that most of us are seriously deficient in. Omega-3 fatty acids are especially important for rejuvenation of our prenatal jing energy and for prevention of many problems of aging. They are needed for building cells, especially the cells of the brain and nervous system, eyes, and circulatory system, including the heart. Omega-3 oils also quell inflammation.

Flax and chia seeds are vegetarian sources of omega-3s. Omega-3s can also be found in "marine lipid" oils—fish oils from salmon, anchovy, sardines, and krill.

Hemp-Seed Oil vs. Flaxseed Oil: A Better Balance

We've all heard of the health benefits of flaxseed oil, an ideal source of omega-3. When you first begin following the Body Ecology Way of Life, it is recommended that you use flaxseed oil to get your omega-3 levels up to where they should be. But eventually you might consider switching to hemp-seed oil. Although flaxseed oil is higher in omega-3, hemp-seed oil provides the ideal ratio of fatty acids—the perfect balance of omega-3, omega-6, and omega-9. Go to **www.manitobaharvest.com** for a good source of hemp-seed oil.

One of our very favorite oils at Body Ecology is derived from the pristine waters of the Marlborough Sounds region of New Zealand, where the unique properties of the ozone layer and intense UV rays cause the highly prized Greenshell mussel ("green-lipped mussel") and other life-forms to develop an unparalleled combination of lipid groups and unique omega-3 polyunsaturated fatty acids—which the native Maori have thrived on for more than 700 years.

Studies show that Greenshell-mussel oil has significant anti-inflammatory properties and can benefit patients with asthma, osteoarthritis, rheumatoid arthritis, asthma, and other inflammatory conditions.

Fat Intolerance

If you have difficulty digesting fats and oils, most likely your liver and/or gallbladder are congested. It is important to begin the process of cleansing your liver, which we'll discuss at greater length later in the book. For now, creating an inner ecosystem of beneficial, fat-digesting microbiota is a must to help break down and assimilate the fats you consume. Fat tolerance will improve as you eat and drink fermented foods and beverages each day.

Symptoms of fat intolerance include pains in the neck and shoulders, spasms in the large and small intestines, feeling tired just after eating, bloating, indigestion, belching, flatulence and/or nausea, upper-right abdominal discomfort, and hard stools. Fat intolerance can be confirmed by a simple urine test or by eliminating fats from your diet for a week and noting any improvement in your digestion and energy.

Fermented foods and enzymes should be taken at every meal to help with digestion of fats.

Keep in mind that combined with animal protein, excessive amounts of fats—even those recommended—delay the secretion of gastric juices. This means those all-American tuna, egg, and chicken salads with heaps of mayo could be contributing to your symptoms of discomfort.

A small amount of organic, unrefined coconut oil, ghee, or red-palm oil used for sautéing shouldn't cause you any discomfort, while salad dressings or heaps of butter on your foods may. (You can find a Body Ecology no-oil salad-dressing recipe at **www.bodyecology.com**.)

Fats and the Principle of Uniqueness

The Body Ecology universal Principle of Uniqueness tells us that we should not compare our own needs for fats and oils with those of others. Each of us is unique. The *quantity* of fat and oil to consume at one time will ultimately depend on the current health of the liver and gallbladder.

And most important, you must ask yourself, "How well do I digest these fats and oils?" Yes, butter can be a valuable fat, but only if it is right for *your* unique body. You are an experiment of one. You have to find out what your body needs at this moment in time, and that need will change constantly. Just tune in to your body and listen. It will communicate to you through signs and symptoms if you eat foods that are *not* right for you.

You can try to determine your own individual need for fats and oils by carefully watching how your body reacts to each one, but *ideally, taking an Essential and Metabolic Fatty Acid Analysis test is best. To find out more about this test, ask your holistically oriented physician.*

The next best thing is to try one fat or oil at a time. When you have not eaten for at least three hours, take a spoonful of the fat or oil, and watch to see how it makes you feel. But again, testing is far more accurate in determining your immediate and individual needs.

Here are a few questions to answer to help determine your unique fat needs:

— **What is your level of activity?** If you are active, you will definitely require more fats in your diet, and you will be able to consume more butter or ghee.

— **Do you live in a cold climate or a hot one?** If you live in a cold climate or in a place with cold seasons, your body will need the extra fat to help you stay warm. Those who retire to Florida or flee to exotic islands will find they can use much less. In fact, they might do best with saturated fat from plants, such as coconut oil and palm oil.

— **Are you a large, big-boned person; or are you small-boned?** Saturated fats are important for healthy bone development. Big bones need more.

— **How's your level of stress?** You may want to increase the amount of butter and ghee in your diet when you are under a lot of stress. (Probably not an issue if you are exploring a tropical island!)

91

— **Are you deficient in the fatty acids found in milk fat?** Have you been avoiding butter for years and been eating margarine instead? At first you may notice that you are actually craving yummy raw butter. Your body truly needs it, so enjoy! You'll soon find that this craving diminishes, and you will be satisfied with less.

— And then, finally, you must deal honestly with these questions: **What is the current condition of your organs, especially your liver and gallbladder? How well do you digest fats today?** Many of us have livers that are very congested and toxic. As we age, the liver also begins to shrink and is supplied with less blood. Ultimately, rejuvenating this organ so that you can benefit from these healthy fats and oils will be necessary.

Fats and the Principle of Balance

When you eat fats, you will want to balance them out with other foods. Fats and oils are slightly expansive and acidic, meaning you'll want to combine them with sea salt, which is strongly contractive and alkaline. Raw daikon, leafy-green salads, apple-cider vinegar, and lemon juice are also great choices because they create balance by helping with the digestion of fats. Ginger, fennel, and tumeric are examples of spices that aid in their digestion as well.

Fats and the Principle of Food Combining

Fats and oils combine well with many foods: grain-like seeds, for example, or meals with animal proteins, including dairy proteins found in milk kefir. Land, ocean, starchy, and fermented vegetables are more delicious with fats and oils.

It's Not Just about Olive Oil Anymore

Many of us are limited by our imaginations when it comes to healthy oils. We may be avoiding the bad oils, such as vegetable and canola oil, but we have made olive oil the *only* oil in our pantry.

While extra-virgin olive oil is an excellent choice for salads, it's not a good idea to cook with it. Why? Under high heat, it burns easily, and when it does, it turns into a toxin. There are certain oils that are better for cooking, because they withstand a higher heat before degenerating. Some we would never want to heat because they lose their *medicinal* qualities. To retain the antioxidants and vitamin E in olive oil, eat it raw.

When you follow the Body Ecology Way of Life, ghee, coconut oil, and red-palm oil are the three oils used to sauté. Raw butter, virgin olive oil, and unrefined seed and nut oils are best drizzled right onto your food or used in salad-dressing recipes. If you want, you can add these to a sauce after it has cooled down a bit or just before eating.

What if you eat out, don't cook, or aren't preparing your food at home every day? There is nothing wrong with taking your needed amount on a spoon. Fish oils also come in capsules.

Documenting the effect that bad fats and oils—coupled with deficiencies of the good ones—have had on us is beyond the scope of this chapter or book, but needless to say, it has been devastating. It's time to turn the fat story around and do it right. It's up to us to correct a serious wrong.

Changing the fats and oils you eat is a good, yet simple, first step. The next chapter will discuss an equally controversial topic today—*protein*.

CHAPTER 9

PROTEIN:
Shedding Light on the Controversy

*Integral to every cell in the body, protein is used
to build and repair tissues, and to make enzymes and
hormones. However, as we age, we must rethink our
protein needs—considering type, quality, and digestibility.*

It's funny how many of us associate some of the most memorable times in our lives with food. One favorite memory of mine was eating with my friends at the Varsity drive-in. The Varsity specialized in chili dogs, kraut dogs, greasy fries, and huge Coca-Colas. I especially loved the kraut dogs—perhaps an early clue to my future love affair with cultured cabbage! When I think of my teen years, I can still remember the smells and warmth of that special time. *Yet if I had only known then what I know now!*

Today, there are a number of compelling reasons why we should change our eating habits—especially with regard to animal protein. The world's total meat supply is increasing at an alarming rate. In 1961, it was estimated at 71 million tons a year. In 2007, that figure had risen to around 284 million tons. Americans continue to eat about eight ounces of meat a day, roughly twice the global average. More meat means more feed, especially corn and soy . . . which not only raises the price, but also exacts a heavy cost on our energy supplies and on our environment.

Eric Schlosser's widely read book *Fast Food Nation* exposes our poorly regulated meat industry and its potential health threats. The problem is not with the animals, but with the way we commercially raise them—in cruel, large-scale confinement facilities. Turning this problem around is one of the most challenging issues facing us today, and it will take a focused effort to tackle it with a compassionate heart.

Is this meant to suggest that you give up meat or other animal proteins such as fish, milk, eggs, and poultry? Perhaps, but the choice will be yours to make. In this chapter you'll find exactly what you need to know to make this decision. Here are six important points to remember:

1. We need protein throughout our lives.

2. Not all proteins are alike.

3. Adequate protein can be obtained from both the animal and plant kingdoms.

4. It is not wise to obtain all your protein from animals. However, if you choose to be a vegetarian, you will have to take great care not to miss out on certain nutrients, including amino acids, minerals, fats, and vitamins, found in animal products.

5. All foods have their positive and negative sides . . . including all protein foods.

6. Proper digestion is crucial to ensure that the value of high-quality protein is not lost.

What Exactly Is a Protein?

If all of the water and fat is removed from the body, 75 percent of what remains is protein. Protein consists of chains of amino acids. There are 22 amino acids that combine to form different types of proteins. Everything from our neurotransmitters, the chemical messengers of our brains; to our organs, blood, bones, hair, and nails is composed of proteins. Nine of the 22 amino acids are called *essential,* and because our bodies can't make them, they must be obtained from the diet. We need to consume proteins or we will be deficient in these essential amino acids.

Your body expends more energy to digest protein than sugars or fats. But unlike sugars, which provide quick energy, protein provides long-lasting energy without an insulin surge (which promotes fat storage). For these reasons, protein can help keep you lean and slender.

The protein in our diets determines the amount of an important hormone in the body called *glucagon,* which helps balance insulin. While insulin can *contribute* to fat storage, glucagon helps prevent it. Body fat, especially abdominal fat, creates inflammation. And low-grade chronic inflammation leads to every disease of aging: diabetes, cardiovascular disease, cancer, Alzheimer's, rheumatoid arthritis, inflammatory bowel disease, and gum disease.

As we age, sarcopenia (muscle wasting) becomes a serious problem. Starting in our early 40s, most of us begin to experience a loss of muscle mass. Those of us entering our seventh decade can expect an even more rapid decline in muscle unless we make changes to our diet, digestion, and way of life. Even if we are physically active, low-grade acidosis, inflammation, and a lack of minerals in the diet will cause our muscles to disappear. Protein helps build muscles that make us look sexier and more youthful.

Sources of Animal Protein

Eggs

Contrary to popular belief, it is the egg *yolk* that is the healthiest part of the egg. Egg yolks are great for your brain, thyroid, and hormones—they contain good fats and are an excellent source of vitamins A and D. They also contain the B vitamin *choline*—the precursor to acetylcholine, an important stimulating neurotransmitter that is deficient in the brains of those with Alzheimer's. Choline also helps convert fats into HDL, the good cholesterol.

This may surprise you if you still believe in an outdated perception that egg yolks raise cholesterol. They do, but you *want* this good cholesterol.

While it is difficult to find them, try to purchase eggs from *pasture-fed* chickens that have not been fed soybeans. In nature, chickens eat worms and bugs for their protein, not soy. They are not vegetarians. Eggs from chickens that eat their natural proteins, live cage-free lives, and are never fed hormones are the very best.

Fish & Shellfish

Oily fish, like salmon, are one of the most preferred animal-protein foods on the Body Ecology program. We recommend having fish at least two or three times per week. Avoid warm-water species, like orange roughy, because preservatives are used when they are caught. Cold-water fish are best, such as salmon, sardines, tuna, and halibut. Salmon and sardines are especially healthy because they are rich in omega-3s.

Meat & Poultry

Meat and poultry, especially from organic, hormone- and anti-biotic-free animals, can be excellent sources of protein for some. While red meat has gotten bad publicity in the past few years, more recent studies are coming out to debunk these myths. Beef, a complete protein, is high in minerals and B vitamins and contains heart-healthy carnitine and coenzyme Q_{10}. Lamb is also an excellent protein, strengthening to many (especially those with blood type B). The important things to remember with regard to beef are *quality* and *preparation.*

Milk Kefir

If dairy works well in your body, this ancient food has long been thought to increase longevity. It is fun, delicious, and very easy to make with Body Ecology's Kefir Starter. Use goat, cow, or sheep milk—raw, if possible. Find a source at: **www.realmilk.com**.

Meat in Moderation

Apart from its global impact on the environment, *excessive* consumption of red-meat protein also exacts a great toll on our health. A study of more than 500,000 middle-aged and older Americans found that those who consumed *more than four ounces of red meat a day* (the equivalent of a small hamburger) were more than 30 percent more likely to die during the ten years in which they were observed, mostly from heart disease and cancer. Sausage, cold cuts, and other processed meats also increased the risk.

At the same time, the study revealed that those who consumed the most white meat (poultry and fish) were about 8 percent *less* likely to die during the study period than those who ate the least. This is because poultry contains more unsaturated fat, which improves cholesterol levels; while fish contains omega-3 fatty acids, which reduce the risk of heart disease.

Researchers stressed that the study results do not mean people should eliminate red meat from their diets entirely, but simply avoid eating it in large amounts and every day. Walter Willett, a nutrition expert at the Harvard School of Public Health, writes: "You can be very healthy being a vegetarian, but you can be very healthy being a non-vegetarian if you keep your red meat intake low."[1]

Sources of Vegetarian Proteins

Nuts & Seeds

Nuts and seeds are nutrient-dense protein/fats, best eaten after soaking 8 to 12 hours to remove the phytic acid that makes them difficult to digest. There are some good reasons not to overdo these foods. Very concentrated sources of protein, nuts and seeds are not only acidic; they are also rich in the amino acid arginine, which often triggers viral outbreaks. If you have herpes or AIDs, avoid them or eat them in very small quantities. Unfortunately, nuts and seeds are also rich in oxalates, which should be avoided, or at least limited, in many people's diets.

Beans

Beans are mostly a carbohydrate combined with some protein. This makes them intrinsically harder to digest. They digest best when combined with land, ocean, and fermented vegetables. To really get the benefits of the protein in beans, they must be soaked for 8 to 24 hours to remove the phytic acid. To minimize the gas-producing effect of beans, soak them for at least 8 hours, and then cook them slowly for 45 minutes in water. Pour off the water and start cooking again. This time, add a strip of the sea vegetable *kombu.* Salt can be added *after* the beans have become soft.

Eating beans only with fresh and cultured veggies in a meal is a big help when it comes to digesting them. Combining beans with a grain such as rice or with a tortilla, as is traditionally done, is not recommended. Beans can also be soaked, sprouted, cooked, and then blended up into a delicious pâté.

Fermented Soybean Foods

The best way to eat beans is to ferment them, and with soybeans, it is absolutely critical to do so. Fermented soy foods such as miso, wheat-free tamari, natto, and tempeh are definitely part of the Body Ecology program and are excellent anti-aging foods.

The phytoestrogens and isoflavones in soybeans have estrogen-like activity and are structurally similar to estrogen. They bind easily to receptor sites on a cell. While unfermented soy foods such as tofu and soy milk have been heavily promoted recently as having significant therapeutic properties for women, most of the claims (breast- and prostate-cancer prevention, reducing cholesterol, and prevention and treatment of postmenopausal symptoms and osteoporosis) have not been confirmed in well-designed clinical trials.

Instead, a more convincing body of research shows that the phytoestrogens being consumed in large quantities in popular *unfermented* soy foods (soy milk, tofu, energy bars, protein shakes, ice cream, yogurt, cheese, hot dogs, and so on) are disrupting the endocrine system. They can cause infertility and can *promote* breast cancer . . . not prevent it. Japanese researcher Hiro Watanbe, an expert in developmental biology and cancer prevention, has shown that *fermented* miso soup helps to dramatically lower the risk of breast cancer and even to reverse it.

If you'd like to learn more about the negative effects of soy, visit the Weston A. Price Foundation website: **westonaprice.org**. Their information is well supported by research.

Natto–for Bones and Beauty

Natto, a traditional food of Japan, has been a staple in that country for more than a thousand years. Sometimes called "vegetable cheese," natto is simply fermented soybeans. Rich in vegetable protein and vitamin B$_{12}$, natto is nourishing, cooling, and antiviral. It has been linked to prevention of cancer, heart attacks, osteoporosis, and obesity. Although these health benefits are often attributed to soy, it's really the *bacteria* in natto that give it its kick. *Bacillus natto* produces various enzymes, vitamins, amino acids, and other nutrients that can only emerge during fermentation.

Under good conditions, natto bacteria can double their numbers in 30 minutes, producing various enzymes that help digestion. *Nattokinase* and *pyrazine* are two enzymes present in natto that prevent or reduce blood clotting, which obstructs the flow of blood and is often the precursor to heart attacks and strokes. Nattokinase is only produced during natto's fermentation process.

Another interesting thing to note about natto is that it has a very high amount of vitamin K, which helps in the formation of our bones. Very few foods contain naturally occurring vitamin K. People with osteoporosis tend to have low amounts, so this is an ideal natural supplement.

And finally, natto has some wonderfully "youthening" cosmetic benefits. Soybeans are high in *lecithin*, a *surfactant* (wetting agent) that balances fat and water in skin cells and on the cell surface. This may explain why Japanese women often have smoother, clearer skin than Europeans and Americans. Natto is also rich in vitamin E, which helps prevent skin damage and keeps us looking young.

Green Drinks with Algae and Cereal Grasses

Look for a whole-food green drink that contains a wide spectrum of beneficial microbiota and beneficial yeast, digestive enzymes, and protein. Examples are Body Ecology's Super Spirulina Plus and our very popular blend called Vitality SuperGreen. Knowing how important it is to alkalize the body and nourish it with easily digested nutrients that assimilate immediately, we've made sure that both of our green protein powders contain fermented ingredients to help heal the digestive tract.

Body Ecology's Grain-like Seeds

Quinoa, millet, buckwheat, and amaranth are protein-rich seeds that are similar to grains and are preferred over rice, wheat, barley, oats, and rye. They should be on your daily menu . . . especially in your evening meal.

Protein Malnourishment

Perhaps you've already accepted that as the years go by your body will become less muscular. Isn't that normal with aging?

Even though we consume twice the global average of animal proteins, protein malnourishment is surprisingly quite common in America. In fact, even our children are protein deficient, yet most consume animal protein every day. *You* may have become protein deficient in childhood even if you were a big "meat eater." Why? Because even from birth, many of us have not been *digesting* the protein we eat.

Protein malnourishment elevates the amount of cortisol in our blood and causes us to feel stressed-out, sleep poorly, and age quickly. A deficiency in protein has other serious negative effects. Our organs fail; thinking, planning, and cognition go on the blink; and the immune system crashes and has difficulty fighting infections. Since our brains, bones, hair, nails, and muscles all rely on protein, they lose their vibrancy—their life force.

Clearly, protein is a vital nutrient, and *eating the right protein foods is vital for combatting aging.* But the $64 million question each of us must now ask is, "If my goal is to add more quality years to my life and eliminate age-related suffering, must I alter the *kind* of protein foods, as well as the *amount*, I eat?" The answer is, without a doubt, yes!

Protein and the Principle of 80/20
(vs. Calorie Restriction)

The word *calorie* is an unpleasant one to many of us who have been dieting for years, and *restriction* is perhaps even more objectionable. Several studies actually suggest that as we age our protein intake needs to be even *higher* than what is currently recommended, and at Body Ecology we agree. We do need *"more" protein* than we are currently consuming, but not more *quantity.* In fact, the secret to pushing back Father Time is to decrease the quantity of protein and add more *quality*—from a *wide variety of sources,* not just animals—and to make sure we digest it better.

Thomas Jefferson probably said it best: "I have lived temperately, eating little animal food, and that not as an aliment, so much as a condiment for the vegetables which constitute my principal diet."[2] A man of many interests, Jefferson was passionate about architecture, gardening, music, wine, and food. Although he never needed to cook his own meals, it is said he frequently collected delicious recipes from chefs and shared them with his friends.

As you envision protein as a "condiment," remember the Principle of 80/20: 80 percent of your serving plate will be land and ocean vegetables; the remaining 20 percent should be animal protein. Always emphasize vegetables—with a focus on adding fermented vegetables, as this is critical to fostering vitality and a healthy inner ecosystem.

By the way, the average life span in Jefferson's day was only 45 years. Born on April 13, 1743, the third U.S. President lived to be 83, dying in 1826. Certainly this man of great intention, intuition, and wisdom had something to tell us.

Animal proteins are potent sources of nutrition. This is one of the main reasons we don't need a large serving at a meal. Even nuts and seeds are concentrated sources of nutrition. Indeed, to truly follow what science is revealing with regard to calorie restriction, we must eat smaller amounts of very *high-quality protein.* And we must discover the proteins that are best for us!

Protein and the Principle of Balance

Animal proteins are *contractive* because of the naturally occurring salt in blood. To create balance, you will feel best if you eat them with more *expansive* foods. For example, a poached salmon or chicken fillet *(contractive)* on top of a big raw salad with a dressing of olive oil and lemon juice or vinegar, plus cultured vegetables *(more expansive)*, creates a very nice balance of ingredients.

Animal protein is also acidic; and since salt, while contracting, is the most alkalizing of all foods, you might have noticed that when you eat certain acidic proteins (fish, eggs, chicken, beef, and even nuts), they taste much more delicious with sea salt. It's your natural instinct to balance the *acid* protein with the very *alkaline* salt.

Nuts and seeds are less contractive than animal proteins. They do not naturally have the salt content of animal foods. You can salt your nuts to make them more alkaline, and they, too, will go nicely in a big raw salad with dressing, plus cultured vegetables.

Chlorella, spirulina, and blue-green algae are excellent vegetarian proteins that have become more and more popular today. While they are alkaline, they have an *expansive,* opening-up quality. Adding a pinch of *contracting* sea salt to a drink containing algae, like Body Ecology's Super Spirulina Plus or E_3Live, can help create that perfect balance. I also recommend adding a pinch of sea salt to a "green veggie smoothie" in the morning, because all those expansive, raw veggies become more balanced with the more contractive sea salt.

Protein and the Principle of Acid/Alkaline

A recent study compared an acidic diet, full of acid-producing proteins and cereal grains, to a diet rich in alkaline-producing fruits and vegetables. The results indicate that metabolic acidosis from the meat-and-grain diet appears to contribute to a reduction in lean tissue mass in older adults. *The alkaline diet favored lean tissue mass.*[3]

If you choose to eat acid-forming proteins, you must balance them with alkaline-forming foods, including small amounts of sour fruits and larger amounts of vegetables from the garden and ocean. If you don't do this, you will rapidly deplete your *chi* or life force.

Protein and the Principle of Food Combining

The meat-and-potatoes meal, characteristic of the standard American diet, is difficult to digest and causes you to gain weight, become acidic, and use up metabolic enzymes, which will age you faster.

To digest animal protein and maximize its benefits, always combine it with non-starchy vegetables from the land and ocean and cultured veggies. For example, combine scrambled eggs with cultured veggies and steamed asparagus.

Nuts and seeds are a *protein/fat,* as is avocado. Dairy foods such as milk kefir and raw cheese are also protein/fats. You could drink a glass of milk kefir and eat some soaked almonds or walnuts. White animal protein should not be eaten with fruits. All protein/fats combine well with members of the acid-fruit family (such as açaí, pomegranate, grapefruit, strawberry, and raspberry). All foods in this protein/fat category can also be combined with vegetables.

Examples:

- Avocado with nuts and seeds and with acid fruits.

- A salad made with romaine lettuce, avocado, soaked and dehydrated sunflower seeds, blueberries, or grapefruit sections. You could even toss in a few cubes of raw cheese (if this protein works for your body).

- A smoothie made with milk kefir, sour Granny Smith apple, celery, zucchini, and stevia to sweeten. A bit of coconut oil would be tasty, too, and a spoonful of chia seeds will add fiber and omega-3 fatty acid.

- All the organic, unrefined oils combine with the proteins mentioned above. In fact, all proteins naturally contain oils. For example, salmon has salmon oil, cod liver has cod-liver oil, walnuts have walnut oil, and hemp seeds have hemp oil. Oil can even be found in algae. The brain-nourishing fatty acid DHA can be obtained from the oil in algae.

The four recommended grain-like seeds—quinoa, millet, amaranth, and buckwheat—are protein/starches. Because of the starch, most people find that these digest best when eaten as the main entrée and combined with starchy and non-starchy vegetables. They are seeds, though, and some people can eat them with animal protein or nuts and seeds. If your digestion is sensitive, this is not recommended. If you must serve a meal with animal protein and a grain, however, these grain-like seeds are a much better choice than traditional protein/grain combinations such as chicken and rice, meatballs with pasta, or eggs with toast and oatmeal.

Protein and the Principle of Uniqueness

Because the Principle of Uniqueness says that no one diet fits all, some of us may feel better and maintain more muscle mass when we eat animal protein. Some of us will feel lighter and more fit if we are vegetarians.

In other words, you will have to decide whether animal protein works in *your* unique body and how much you should be eating each day. (Or perhaps only several times per week?)

The Body Ecology Way, with its 7 Universal Principles; excellent-quality fats and oils; and wide array of fermented foods and liquids, protein powders, and grain-like seeds, can also enhance the diet of any vegetarian or vegan who has chosen a non-carnivore way of life. You would then also have the benefits of a gluten-free, sugar-free diet. This will help you maintain the important anti-aging, acid/alkaline balance of your blood.

The best place to begin is by asking yourself the right questions, educating yourself, and seeking out a source for reliable testing. You might consider consulting with a Body Ecology Coach or scheduling a visit to a health-care professional who knows the Body Ecology way.

Start paying attention to *your* body. Maybe you'll find that where you live right now requires you to eat more animal protein and fats. It's harder to eat only raw foods when you live in a cold climate, because they cool the body and provide no warmth. They work well in warmer climates, like the Southwest, Florida, Hawaii, and California, however . . . where you'll notice most raw foodists reside.

What's your age? A growing baby will not have the same nutritional needs as someone in his or her 70s.

What's happening with your own hormones? Did you eat a lot of acidic foods such as meat, pasta, and ice cream as a child and as an adult . . . and are you now experiencing hot flashes and low libido in your 40s? An acid-forming diet will wreak havoc with your hormones, burning out your endocrine system quickly and causing you to age.

And very important, what are you *digesting* right now? Undigested food becomes another toxin in your digestive tract, so how you prepare what you eat so that you can digest it will be fundamental.

Being Vegetarian or Vegan the Body Ecology Way

The Body Ecology way of eating is mostly plant based but not necessarily vegetarian. Millions of us feel stronger and more grounded when we eat animal foods. We also have a powerful emotional and even genetic attachment to them. Not only have we grown up eating them every day, but as a species we've been doing so for thousands of years, and our cells and our genes are familiar with them. They simply seem comforting and natural to us.

That said, some of us prefer to be "vegetarian" while still consuming animal products such as dairy foods and eggs. This arrangement feels good because the animal has not been killed, yet the vegetarian is obtaining important nutrients available only in animal sources of food.

Many of us who have tried a raw, vegan diet feel lighter and more energetic. Others of us find we cannot digest raw vegetables. When you embark on a vegan or raw-foods diet, you might thrive for a certain period of time—say, one day, one week, a month, or several years—on this lighter fare. This is because it is right for your *unique* body at this point in your life. But then maybe you notice you're beginning to look older, or your spine is developing a curve. Your teeth and gums may have started to deteriorate, and you can't carry on a focused conversation with your accountant. These conditions can be related to protein deficiency. Please don't be so committed to being a vegan that you deprive your body of nutrients it needs.

An excellent source of omega-3 can be obtained from a fish-oil supplement. There are other important nutrients in animal protein. Cod-liver oil, butter, ghee, and egg yolks provide vitamins A and D. Vegetarians can become deficient in B_{12} and important amino acids such as tyrosine and taurine. Full-spectrum amino-acid supplements are available but should be unnecessary if you are eating the right vegetarian protein foods and digesting them properly. Supplements are great, but there is nothing as effective as well-digested food. You might also consider adding Body Ecology's Super Spirulina Plus powder to your diet, as this is an excellent source of folic acid and B_{12}.

Be watchful . . . and when you see symptoms of low energy, anxiety, spaciness, tooth decay, hormonal imbalances, and loss of sexual desire, it may be time to add in more grounding animal foods and/ or animal fats such as butter, ghee, cod-liver oil, egg yolks, or even raw-milk kefir.

How to Prepare Animal Protein for Ideal Digestion

To digest protein, you must have strong "digestive fire." This means adequate amounts of digestive enzymes in your stomach and small intestine. Hydrochloric acid (HCl), pepsin, and pancreatic enzymes (found in the small intestine) that digest protein and fats are often inadequate or nonexistent. Ironically, when you are too acidic and deficient in minerals, your stomach will not produce enough stomach acid—creating a vicious cycle: low stomach acid equals low minerals; then low minerals equal low stomach acid.

If you find you feel stronger and more grounded when you eat animal proteins but have weak digestion, then you must find ways to prepare these foods so that they are easy to digest.

— **Prepare as a puree.** "Blenderize" your animal proteins such as chicken or fish into a pâté (like baby food). Salmon pâté can be a tasty delicacy.

— **Prepare savory stocks.** Prepare only the *broth* of the animal (fish, chicken, or lamb broth). *Note:* Be sure to remove the cooked saturated fat from your broth before you eat it.

— **Dine on rare, raw, and fermented food.** Indigenous people around the world instinctively knew to eat a portion of their animal protein such as fish, milk, or meat either raw or fermented. In fact, sausage is traditionally a fermented food. When you cook animal proteins, you denature the protein, and they become impossible to digest. Undigested animal protein is simply another toxin in your gut. Too much over a long time can lead to cancer.

— **Serve fermented foods and liquids at each meal.** Including fermented foods in your diet—especially having cultured veggies and/ or young coconut kefir with your protein meals—is a must. Cultured veggies are full of enzymes that enhance the digestion of proteins. A lovely wineglass full of young coconut kefir or InnergyBiotic is a great digestive aid. Sip it slowly as you eat your meal.

Now that you know the importance of cutting back on the amount of animal protein in your diet, what foods will you need to embrace more of to restore your prenatal jing? The next chapter showcases one of the most critical food pillars in the Body Ecology program—*vegetables*.

From the Physician's Desk

The price of a high-protein diet . . . is it worth it?

It has been well documented that high-protein diets are a primary cause of increased loss of calcium from bones, which leads to thinning and loss of bone (osteopenia and osteoporosis). Alarming data reveal that 50 percent of women above the age of 55 have this problem.

The overconsumption of protein and other acid-producing foods, such as grains, sugars, alcohol, and salt, increases both the acid load and acid production in the body. To make matters worse, the under-consumption of alkaline-producing foods—namely, vegetables, fruits, and minerals (especially potassium, magnesium, and calcium in the citrate and bicarbonate forms)—compounds the problem, creating even more acidosis. The breakdown of calcium phosphate from bone is the body's way of correcting the acid/alkaline imbalance. So, the bones get thinner, the phosphate buffers the increased acid in the blood, and the high calcium, which leaves the body via the urine, can create kidney stones and/or greatly stress the kidneys. In addition, the higher calcium in the presence of acidosis can be deposited in areas of inflammation such as arteries, tendons, ligaments, joints, muscles, and even the brain. This is known as *ectopic calcification,* or the laying down of calcium where it doesn't belong.

A recent study showed how easily and quickly this bone-loss process can begin, even in women as young as 22 to 39. In other words, premenopausal women on a standard American high-protein diet can be putting themselves at significant risk of premature bone loss, which accumulates over time. The researchers took 39 healthy premenopausal women, consuming their typical higher-protein diet, and reduced it to .8 grams of protein per kilogram of body weight for only a two-week period. The lab tests at the end of the study period showed some surprising results:

- Decreases in urine- and blood-nitrogen levels
- Decreases in renal-acid secretion
- Decreases in calcium and bone-loss markers in the urine

These data show that even in a two-week period, eating a little less protein and a lot more vegetables, fruits, and minerals can modify this chronic and dangerous problem.[i]

— *Leonard Smith, M.D.*

---

[i] B. Avery Ince, Ellen J. Anderson, and Robert M. Neer, "Lowering Dietary Protein to U.S. Recommended Dietary Allowance Levels Reduces Urinary Calcium Excretion and Bone Resorption in Young Women," *The Journal of Clinical Endocrinology & Metabolism,* Vol. 89, No. 8 (2004): 3801–3807.

CHAPTER 10

VEGETABLES:
For Vitamins and Minerals

Processed foods and sweets have spoiled our taste buds, causing us to lose our instinctive fondness for natural, whole foods such as vegetables. And yet vegetables come in so many varieties, flavors, and colors—and they have so many incredible health benefits—they deserve to be billed as <u>superfoods</u>.

Most of us can remember the famous comic-strip character Popeye the Sailor, who first surfaced in 1929. In the 1930s Paramount began to release cartoon shorts, which became syndicated for television in the 1950s.[1] It was then that Popeye's considerable strength became forever tied to his heroic consumption of spinach.

What people didn't find out until much later was that Popeye's creator had read a study published in the late 1870s that contained a misprint.[2] The article erroneously stated that spinach had ten times its actual iron content. (The real iron content is on par with most other vegetables.) But by then the Popeye mythology was well established.

During the '30s, Popeye's popularity helped boost sales of spinach nationwide, and a 33 percent increase in spinach consumption was reported. The spinach-growing community of Crystal City, Texas, actually erected a statue in tribute to the iconic hero. Popeye's love interest was *Olive Oyl,* and their adopted baby boy was named *Swee'pea.* Famous expressions like "I yam what I yam" quickly endeared Popeye to his fans. Perhaps all of these many references to produce prompted mothers everywhere to say to their offspring: "Eat your vegetables!"

Mother certainly knew best, as vegetables are nutritional power-houses that keep us active, mentally alert, and forever young.

Vegetables Are Youth Enhancing

Vegetables from the land and the ocean might be called nature's most perfect anti-aging foods—rich in the vitamins and minerals needed to sustain and vitalize your body. A wide variety of beautifully colored vegetables should comprise 80 percent of your diet. Easy to digest, they are nutrient-dense but low in calories; and because they are alkaline, they help fight the acidic environment that causes inflammation, yeast overgrowth, and viruses, which tend to worsen as we age.

New research on vegetables and aging shows that on measures of mental sharpness, vegetables give you an edge. In a study funded by the National Institute on Aging, 2,000 Chicago-area men and women were tested at the end of a six-year period. Older people who ate more than two servings of vegetables daily appeared about five years younger at the end of the study than those who ate few or no vegetables. In addition, people who ate more than two servings of vegetables a day had about 40 percent less mental decline than those who ate few or no vegetables.

Leafy-green vegetables such as spinach, kale, collards, mustard greens, and kohlrabi appear to be especially powerful, as they contain significant amounts of minerals and the antioxidant vitamins C, A, and E. When paired with healthy fats such as olive oil, they are even more effective, as these oils help the body absorb the antioxidants. The same study also found that people who ate lots of vegetables tended to be more physically active. This in turn has a positive effect on brain acuity and memory.[3]

Vegetables Are Powerful Detoxifiers

In recent years, a lot of scrutiny has been given to the "cruciferous" family of vegetables. Cabbage, broccoli, Brussels sprouts, cauliflower, kale, collards, and bok choy are frequent favorites in our Body Ecology kitchens. They all have natural cancer-fighting substances (*isothiocyanates* and *indoles*) that help regulate and improve the 2:16 hydroxyestrone ratio, a proven predictor of hormone-related cancers such as breast and prostate. In short, a normal 2:16 ratio means less cancer risk.

Other green vegetables, including mustard greens, watercress, and Swiss chard, are excellent sources of *carotenoids,* which protect against eye diseases such as macular degeneration. They are also good sources of beta-carotene, another cancer fighter.

You might not be aware of this, but healthy plants actually do defend themselves by producing a variety of bad-tasting substances that cause them to be toxic and inedible to animals and insects. Some, however, contain toxins that offer bitter or other pleasingly complex tastes that appeal to us humans. Most of these plant toxins are *phytonutrients,* important detoxifiers that help our bodies get rid of spent hormones and environmental poisons.

It's important to note that phytonutrients are more abundant in *organically grown* vegetables because, unlike conventionally grown produce that is protected from insects by spraying with pesticides, organic cultivation preserves the natural defenses of the plant, allowing the phytonutrients to survive. Just a few of these phytonutrient-rich plants include: garlic, ginger, onions, rosemary, green tea, wasabi, and the cruciferous vegetables (as well as blueberries, black currants, and pomegranates).[4]

Land Vegetables

As you start to increase the *amount* of vegetables you eat at each meal—yes, even at breakfast—you'll also want to include a wide *variety*. There is an amazing array of vegetables available today. You'll see that their colors, textures, and shapes add excitement to any meal.

Leafy-green vegetables grow above ground (for example, turnip greens, kale, collards, and beet greens) and are rich in chlorophyll from the sun. Not only do they help cleanse your blood, but they are also excellent sources of calcium and iron. *Eat them at least once a day.*

Root vegetables, which grow underground (for example, carrots, onions, daikon, and turnips), are slightly more contracting in nature and provide strength and winter warmth. Some root vegetables naturally contain more sugars, such as beets, parsnips, sweet potatoes, and yams. If you have an inflammation-causing infection (yeast or virus) or high blood sugar, then *fermenting* these nutrient-rich root vegetables (when you make a cultured-vegetable blend) is a great way to eliminate the sugar.

Low in calories and high in fiber, vegetables are excellent foods for maintaining healthy intestines.

In a nutshell, from the Body Ecology perspective, you almost can't eat "too many" vegetables. It is highly recommended that your diet consist of 80 percent vegetables (or about seven to ten servings per day)—prepared in many delicious ways.

Recommended Non-starchy Vegetables

Arugula	Collard greens
Asparagus	Corn (if raw)
Bamboo shoots	Cucumbers
Beet greens	Daikon
Bok choy	Dandelion greens
Broccoli	Endive
Brussels sprouts	Escarole
Burdock root	Fennel
Cabbage	Garlic
Carrots (if raw)	Green beans
Cauliflower	Jicama
Celeriac	Kale
Celery	Kohlrabi
Celery root	Lamb's-quarters
Chives	Leeks

Mustard greens

Okra

Onions

Parsley

Radishes (red)

Red bell pepper
   (in small quantities)

Scallions

Shallots

Spinach

Swiss chard

Turnips (and greens)

Watercress

Yellow bell peppers
   (in small quantities)

Yellow squash

Zucchini

Recommended Starchy Vegetables

Artichokes (and Jerusalem artichokes)

Carrots (mildly starchy when cooked)

Corn (fresh on or off the cob, mildly starchy when cooked)

Peas (English)

Red-skin potatoes

Shiitake and other wild mushrooms

Winter squash (acorn, butternut, or buttercup)

New Thoughts on Some Old Standbys

There are many other vegetables besides the ones recommended here that you might want to experiment with, not only for flavor, but simply for expanding your "treasure chest" of nature's gifts for reversing your biological age.

We have found that *a few vegetables are best not eaten at all*, depending upon the health status of the individual. Examples are:

- **Cooked beets, parsnips, sweet potatoes, and yams:** These vegetables are too high in natural sugars unless cultured.

- **Eggplant, bell peppers, and tomatoes:** Members of the nightshade family of vegetables, they often irritate the nervous system, and some believe they aggravate arthritis. People who are highly sensitive or hyperactive should not eat them. Others can eat them in moderation. Green bell peppers are red peppers picked at an early stage and are very difficult to digest. Our recipes only use red peppers and in small amounts. Tomatoes may be tolerated occasionally, in season, with a green salad. When cooked, they become even more acid forming than when eaten raw.

- **Russet and Yukon Gold potatoes:** These are very high in sugar. Red-skin potatoes, also called "new potatoes," are lower in sugar. Remember: Each of us is unique; and the sugars in potatoes may be fine for you, especially if you eat them in a meal with something fermented— for example, a juice glass of young coconut kefir or a serving of cultured vegetables. These fermented foods contain the microbiota to digest the sugars. Potatoes also belong to the nightshade family (see above), so you may want to avoid them if they seem to cause joint stiffness and arthritic symptoms.

- **Indoor, tray-grown wheatgrass:** Really a long sprout, it is too sweet and expansive for many.

- **Mung bean and other sprouts:** These usually have mold on them. Broccoli sprouts, however, are an excellent food.

Vegetables can be labor-intensive and time-consuming to prepare, which is why restaurants offer so few of them on their menus! But they can actually save time in the long run if you cook up larger batches so that they last for a couple of days. For example, make big pots of soups or stews that contain a variety of vegetables. Twice a week, cook dark green, leafy vegetables and ocean vegetables, but eat them all week long. Having lettuce washed and ready to go in the refrigerator will also save you time.

Oxalates—What Popeye Didn't Know

Those who suffer from leaky gut syndrome, edema, autism, chronic obstructive pulmonary disease (COPD), asthma, kidney stones, or vulvodynia, or have difficulty digesting fat may find they need to consider a *low-oxalate diet*. *Oxalates* are substances that are found naturally in the leaves, stems, and roots of many of the most nutritious vegetables. Generally, oxalates are not harmful, because the microbiota in the gut metabolize them, and they leave our bodies through our stools. But if you have destroyed your intestinal microbiota with antibiotics, with stress, or with a high-sugar diet and have never known the importance of establishing a healthy inner ecosystem, you can have oxalate issues.

Until recently, the list of valuable foods high in oxalates included strawberries, blueberries, quinoa, kale, collards, mustard greens, parsley, leeks, celery, green beans, summer squash . . . and yes, even Popeye's favorite, *spinach*. I say "until recently" because we now know that the oxalate content of food can vary considerably between plants of the same species. Differences in climate, soil quality, state of ripeness, or even the part of the plant analyzed will give a different oxalate rating, so that old list is now being reevaluated.

Our bodies always contain oxalates and routinely convert other substances, such as vitamin C, into them. They are also important for managing calcium in the body. Oxalates are not usually absorbed from the gut, but an inflamed, permeable, "leaky" gut lining will allow them to pass through. In the bloodstream, the oxalates bind with calcium, then crystallize. These crystals lodge in weak tissues and cause even more inflammation and pain.

Avoiding foods high in oxalates at least temporarily until the gut problem is solved is a must if you have any of the conditions mentioned previously. You should especially avoid some of the worst offenders—coffee, chocolate, nuts, spinach, black tea, and all wheat products.

Cabbage–the Great Cancer Killer

Diets high in cruciferous vegetables—cabbage, kale, bok choy, and collards—result in fewer instances of certain cancers, including lung, colon, liver, breast, ovarian, and bladder. This may be because cruciferous vegetables optimize your cells' ability to detoxify and cleanse. Not only are cruciferous vegetables high in *isothiocyanates* (powerful anticarcinogens), but scientists have also found them to stimulate phase II enzymes, special liver enzymes that neutralize and dispose of toxins that cause cancer. *Cabbage is particularly beneficial.* High in anticancer compounds called *glucosinolates,* cabbage has shown very good results in lowering the risk of breast cancer.

For example, Polish women consume three times the amount of cabbage that American women do. The rate of breast cancer rose threefold when these women immigrated to the United States.[i] And when you ferment cabbage (sauerkraut), the benefits really skyrocket. Researchers have found that fermented cabbage is healthier than raw or cooked cabbage and more effective at fighting cancer.[ii]

Fermenting releases enzymes that decompose glucosinolate, breaking it down into more accessible isothiocyanates. In addition to these anticancer compounds, fermented cabbage is a good source of minerals, vitamin C, and fiber; and is easier to digest.

---

[i] Jeff Minerd, "AACR: A Diet High in Cabbage May Help Prevent Breast Cancer," University of Pennsylvania School of Medicine, October 31, 2005, **http://www .medpagetoday.com/HematologyOncology/BreastCancer/2035** (accessed 12/14/09).

[ii] Marja Tolonen, Marianne Taipale, Britta Viander, Juha-Matti Pihlava, Hannu Korhonen, and Eeva-Liisa Ryhänen, MTT Agrifood Research Finland, Food Research, FIN-31600 Jokioinen, Finland, *J. Agric. Food Chem.,* 50 (2002): 6798–6803.

It was once believed that dietary calcium should also be avoided. Not so. There is now plenty of research showing that calcium is actually needed when ingesting oxalate-rich foods. The calcium helps decrease the absorption of the oxalates. Prebiotics such as chicory inulin (found in Body Ecology's EcoBloom) will also help increase absorption of calcium from the colon.

For people sensitive to oxalates, keeping the total amount consumed per day below 40 to 60 milligrams is a must. Do not eat spinach, for example, because, when *steamed,* it contains about 697 milligrams in just a half cup . . . and even more if eaten raw. A low-oxalate food would have only 5 milligrams per serving and a medium-oxalate food would have less than 10 . . . so steamed spinach, at 697 milligrams, is not recommended.

(*Note:* Whenever you *boil* vegetables, a significant amount of oxalates is lost in the cooking water. *Steaming* is not as effective as boiling and, depending on the food, may or may not lower them. The cooking water or "pot liquor" should not be eaten, as it does contain the oxalates.)

Here's some good news. Until recently it was believed that *all* green vegetables were high in oxalates. Fortunately, this is not true.

Recently, Susan Owens, who heads up an excellent website on oxalates (**www.lowoxalate.info**), began working with Liebman Lab in Wyoming to test each plant food for its oxalate content. They were quite pleased to find that not *all* greens are high in oxalates after all. After carefully testing each individual food, they learned that boiled kale (4.9 milligrams per half cup), boiled mustard greens (3.2 milligrams per half cup), and boiled collards (8.7 milligrams per half cup) were surprisingly *low* in oxalates.

So if you believe you may be sensitive to oxalates and want to avoid high-oxalate foods, it is important to obtain the most recent oxalate rating on each food (updated on Owens's website). As Owens cautions, "We can no longer make generalizations about oxalate content in foods. Research is now showing us that there are some foods in every category that are high in oxalates and plenty that are also low in oxalates."[5]

We don't want to miss out on these important foods, so what can we do if we are sensitive to oxalates?

Once again, fermentation to the rescue!

If you feel you are sensitive to oxalates—or if kidney stones, COPD, and asthma run in your family—at first limit high-oxalate foods. But don't stop there. Ultimately, you must heal your intestines and create a vibrant, hardy inner ecosystem teeming with a variety of beneficial bacteria. Beneficial microbes in your gut not only keep it healthy, but certain strains are proving to be effective at eating up or degrading oxalates. The most effective oxalate eater is a bacterium called *Oxalobacter formigenes.* This bacterium is not currently available as a supplement, but hopefully will be someday.

However, other beneficial bacteria are proving to be effective oxalate eaters. *Bifidus infantis* (sold under the name of Life Start by Natren) is quite effective at eating oxalates. *L. plantarum* (found abundantly in Body Ecology's cultured vegetables) and *L. breve* do so but appear to be modest eaters, and *L. acidophilus* and *L. thermophilus* were also quite good. *B. infantis* grew rapidly in the presence of oxalates, as did *L. plantarum* and *L. brevis.* This is important, as the microbiota must grow well in the presence of oxalates to be useful to us.[6]

Raw vs. Cooked Vegetables

A growing number of people believe that when you cook vegetables, you destroy or minimize their nutritional content. In fact, the raw-food, vegan diet proposed by Ann Wigmore decades ago has been enjoying a resurgence in popularity for about ten years now.

However, among those in the know, this way of eating is heading out of style. It is not balanced, and nutritional deficiencies often result when only raw foods are eaten for years. Lately, some of the most well-known "thought leaders" in the raw, vegan movement are "coming out of the closet" to say that raw/vegan as a way of life (100 percent of the time, for an extended period) is *not* the way to go after all. Their courage and honesty to admit this is really admirable.

Yes, eating raw foods can be good for you . . . and has many benefits, but raw is not always the right choice. In fact, eating *all* raw can be harmful to some, as raw foods can be difficult to digest and "chilling" for the thyroid (which needs good fats, lots of minerals, and warming foods).

Vegetables and the Principle of Balance

As you learn more about the Body Ecology Way of Life and master the 7 Principles, in the end you will once again see that it all comes down to a matter of balance. Think variety . . . and think *raw, cooked,* and *cultured* when you plan your meals. We humans have been given our creative brains and incredible intelligence to devise wonderfully nourishing, healing, and even "youthening" foods by preparing them in a variety of ways and mastering the art of balance.

How Destructive Is Cooking . . . Really?

Because everything in this wonderful world we live in has both a positive and a negative side, there is also a positive and a negative side to cooking foods. And there is a positive and negative side to eating them raw.

Well-respected food scientist Shirley Corriher provides additional insight on this subject in her excellent book *CookWise: The Hows and Whys of Successful Cooking,* where she shows how science can be applied to traditional cooking.

Here's what she had to say about cooking vegetables:

"You would expect different cooking methods to result in different losses of nutrients, and there are differences—more so with vitamins than with minerals—but not as much as you might think. The mineral loss is relatively small (5 to 10 percent) no matter how the vegetable is cooked. On the other hand, the loss of vitamins varies somewhat, but many vegetables lose only 20 percent or less no matter what the cooking method. This is not to say, however, that there isn't great variability in the nutrient content, because there are very large differences in nutrient content before cooking."[i]

There can be a huge difference in the nutrient content of one carrot over another. The variety the carrot belongs to, the growing conditions, the time it is harvested (was it allowed to reach maturity?), and how it was cared for once it was harvested (was it refrigerated immediately?) all greatly influence the nutritional content.

For example, you can lose as much as 50 percent of your vitamin C in 24 hours by not keeping your food refrigerated. Vitamin C content will be lower if you are purchasing your food from a store with poor refrigeration.

Corriher also states that plants will have a greater amount of vitamin C and beta-carotene when they are grown in more sunlight.

Here are a few more tips to create enzyme-rich, nutrient-dense meals:

- If vegetables are cooked in water, the minerals and the water-soluble vitamins (vitamin C and some B vitamins) will be lost into the cooking water. To solve this problem, either do not

- cook them in water or use the broth from the vegetable water in your recipe so that you obtain those nutrients.

- If you cook your vegetables in a way that heats them to a temperature above approximately 105° F, certain nutrients such as vitamin C and thiamine are destroyed. Does this mean cooking is bad? Absolutely not. It means a wise person makes sure that the lost nutrient is supplied elsewhere in the meal.

- Lost enzymes can easily be obtained in a well-balanced Body Ecology meal. Simply sip on a small wineglass of a probiotic liquid, and of course, eat cultured veggies. For example, adding a few spoonfuls of cultured veggies made with cabbage would make up for any vitamin C lost in cooking. These fermented foods and beverages supply trillions of enzymes, enhance digestion, and provide beneficial microbiota. As explained in Chapter 6, they also provide the "sour taste" that every meal should have to make it really satisfying. Sour is the taste that takes away cravings for sugar and carbs as well.

- Cooking vegetables whole, in their skin, helps prevent some nutrient loss.

---

[i]Shirley O. Corriher, *CookWise: The Hows and Whys of Successful Cooking* (New York: HarperCollins Publishers, Inc., 1997): 353.

Vegetables, Seasons, and the Principle of 80/20

Body Ecology recommends that you practice the 80/20 Principle by eating 80 percent of your vegetables raw and 20 percent cooked during the hot summer months when cooked foods are less desirable, and simply reversing this during the cold winter months. If you live in a hot climate, you might want to eat more raw vegetables year-round.

Raw-Vegetable Smoothies vs. Vegetable Juices

Raw-vegetable *smoothies* . . . especially for breakfast . . . can bring outstanding nutritional qualities to your anti-aging diet. They are cleansing and healing and require less energy to digest than most foods. Regular consumption of veggie smoothies is highly recommended for everyone.

Vegetable smoothies are preferred to vegetable *juices* on the Body Ecology program because they include the vegetable *fiber.* Without it, the vegetables are assimilated into your bloodstream too quickly and make your body acidic. In a smoothie, the fiber is "blenderized" but still there, helping improve detoxification and elimination.

When you wake up each morning after a long night's sleep, your body tends to be dehydrated, too acidic, and too contracted, so vegetable smoothies are a superior alternative to breakfast cereals. Also, consider a day of "fasting" on them to give your liver and digestive tract a rest.

Body Ecology Smoothie Tips

1. While your smoothie will have a base of filtered water, I suggest that approximately 30 percent of the total vegetable content be celery. This is a rich source of natural sodium, ideal for recharging and building your adrenals. Zucchini, romaine lettuce, a few sprigs of cilantro and mint, and cucumber are some favorites to include in your starter base. Then add any of the other ingredients mentioned below.

2. A small *sour* apple, such as a Granny Smith, or other *sour* fruit or juice—pomegranate, unsweetened açaí, cranberry, or black currant—works well in a green smoothie to make it more delicious. However, most fruits and very sweet vegetables such as carrots, beets, and fennel are best avoided.

3. Smoothies should be consumed alone on an empty stomach. Allow 30 to 45 minutes for them to be digested before eating solid foods. They are very filling.

4. Organic, unrefined fats and oils can be added to your smoothie recipe. Examples are: hemp-, pumpkin-,

and flaxseed oil; macadamia, walnut, and pine-nut oil; coconut and avocado oil; and raw cream.

5. "Chewing" your smoothie by holding it in your mouth and mixing it with saliva allows the digestion process to begin, which makes a big difference.

6. Chia seeds can add even more fiber. Body Ecology's EcoBloom is both a fiber and a prebiotic that helps feed the friendly microbiota to help them grow stronger and colonize more effectively. It also helps with absorption of calcium.

7. Blend in extra proteins from one of the following: un-denatured whey-protein concentrate; milk kefir; yogurt; coconut milk; Body Ecology's Vitality SuperGreen; Super Spirulina Plus, our fermented protein powder; or a scoop of raw nut or seed butter.

8. Vanilla flavoring and non-caloric sweeteners such as stevia or Lakanto are nice additions if you like your smoothie on the sweet side. A pinch of sea salt helps create balance. I love potassium-rich Hawaiian sea salt.

9. And please don't forget a splash of your favorite probiotic. Add either a probiotic powder or a probiotic liquid, such as Body Ecology's Young Coconut Kefir, InnergyBiotic, Dong Quai, or CocoBiotic.

Ocean Vegetables

For many Westerners, ocean vegetables (also called sea vegetables) may be a new food. Don't let the idea of eating seaweed put you off. These anti-aging vegetables are wonderfully rejuvenating and so high in nutritional value that they are considered a must. You may need to educate yourself a little about them, but soon you will come to love the taste.

Ocean vegetables are really algae colonies or single-cell organisms that grow on rocks or other ocean surfaces. They are red, blue, green, and black; thrive only in clean water; and are harvested like land vegetables. After harvesting, they are dried and packaged. Ocean vegetables contain more protein and amino acids (building blocks of protein) than beans. They are a good source of iodine, carotene, enzymes, and fiber—and high in vitamins A, C, E, B_1, B_2, B_6, and B_{12}. You may be most familiar with the ocean vegetable *nori* from eating sushi, but there are many other varieties, including *kelp, dulse, hijiki, wakame,* and *arame* (see next page for more information on each type).

Ocean vegetables have many benefits, which include:

- Helping prevent aging—in areas of Japan, where ocean vegetables are harvested, women in their 60s often look as if they are in their 30s

- Regulating the thyroid and providing it with a significant source of iodine

- Enhancing and prolonging the color of hair and lips

- Controlling the growth of pathogenic bacteria, fungi, and viruses

- Providing an abundance of easily digested minerals and trace elements lacking in our diets today

- Restoring and maintaining proper acid/alkaline balance in the body

- Strengthening the nervous and immune systems

- Removing radioactive elements, carcinogens, and even environmental pollutants

- Providing calcium and large amounts of chlorophyll

- Keeping the body more alkaline

- Supplying the colon, liver, thyroid, and adrenals with minerals needed to function properly (ocean vegetables are high in mineral salts, and the "toning" effect on the colon can help resolve constipation)

A Selection of Ocean Vegetables

There are many wonderful ways to incorporate ocean vegetables into your diet. They can be added to soups, sauces, and salads, or dried into snacks.

— **Dulse.** High in iron and great for energy and brain food, dulse can be eaten straight from the package. It has a salty taste and used to be served as a snack in taverns in the early 1900s. While tavern owners hoped that the salty taste would increase patrons' desire for alcohol, they didn't know that dulse also balanced alcohol's effect of leaching minerals from the body.

— **Nori.** Typically used to make sushi in Japanese restaurants, nori is a great snack food because of its mild, nutty, salty taste. You can pass a sheet quickly over the stove burner until it changes color from black to green—or buy it already toasted. Eaten alone, enjoyed in sushi, used as a wrap for grains or veggies, or shredded and added to salads . . . there are many ways to experiment with nori. It contains 28 percent protein, and of all the ocean vegetables, it is one of the highest in vitamins. It also provides calcium, manganese, copper, iron, zinc, and fluoride.

— **Kombu.** An excellent medicinal stock for soups or cooking grains, kombu has several benefits and has been known to counteract high blood pressure. It is high in calcium, iodine, potassium, and vitamins A and C. Kombu contains glutamic acid, which can soften food and add flavor. It can also be cooked with beans to improve their digestibility and reduce their flatulence-producing properties. If you dry strips of kombu at a low temperature in your oven, they become crispy like bacon and make a great snack. You can also use kombu as soup stock. Simply simmer a strip or two in springwater for an hour and add vegetables such as cabbage, carrots, and onions to the broth for a quick and refreshing soup.

— **Wakame.** Tender and sweet tasting, wakame has many of the same benefits as kombu. It is high in calcium and vitamins B and C. Wakame is used in Eastern medicine for its benefits to the skin, hair, intestines, blood, and reproductive organs.

— **Agar.** Derived from red seaweed, agar is a natural gelatin that is superior to animal gelatin. It is used to create delicious aspics, puddings, and gelatin desserts. Agar lubricates the digestive tract and has mild laxative properties. It is a source of vitamins, calcium, phosphorus, iron, and iodine.

— **Arame.** An excellent source of protein, arame has a sweet, nutty flavor and is a good choice for those new to ocean vegetables. It can be tossed into a salad after soaking, with no need for cooking. It can also be added to stir-fries and other cooked meals. A rich source of iodine and iron, it contains calcium and potassium and has beneficial properties to counteract high blood pressure.

— **Hijiki.** With a mild salty or "fishy" flavor, hijiki is the ocean vegetable that is highest in minerals, and it is also known to counteract high blood pressure. A great source of iron, calcium, protein, and trace elements, hijiki makes a wonderful addition to soups and salads.

Just like fermented foods, there are many varieties of ocean vegetables to try, so have fun experimenting! If you seek convenience, consider an ocean-vegetable supplement in order to get the healthy benefits of these superfoods.

Ocean Vegetables and Your Thyroid

With so many people today experiencing thyroid issues, adding ocean vegetables to the diet can be very healing. Thyroid problems can lead to obesity, excessive thinness, hypertension, flatulence, stubborn cases of constipation, fatigue, nervousness, depression, headaches, and neck and shoulder pain.

Ocean vegetables, rich in iodine and other minerals, are very medicinal for the thyroid. Within a week or two of eating them every day, you should notice that you feel calmer in both mind and body. Ocean vegetables reduce tension, help you cope with stress, and enable your body to store vitality and energy.

The thyroid also influences the health of the ovaries, prostate gland, and pyloric valve. It's common to have problems with the pylorus, the valve at the end of the stomach, which must open and close at the correct time to allow food into the small intestine. If you suffer from indigestion, it's especially important to eat ocean vegetables.

Fermented Vegetables and Juices

One of the many bonuses of eating vegetables that have been fermented is that they enhance our taste buds. The flavors in foods will be stronger and more satisfying.

Fermented vegetables and veggie juices are sour; and when you eat them, you can really taste the natural sweetness in other foods such as carrots, beets, and onions. The sugars found in processed foods will seem unpleasantly and artificially sweet, so you can naturally avoid them. Fermenting vegetables also increases their bioavailability, meaning more of the nutritional benefits are getting through.

And if weight is an issue for you and/or you find yourself with constant daily cravings for carbohydrates, alcohol, drugs, and nicotine, you may notice your desire for such destructive substances soon disappears when fermented foods are eaten. At Body Ecology, we would welcome more research on this important property of fermented foods and drinks.

Go Organic and Buy Local

Organic vegetables are preferred, whenever possible, for their higher mineral content and lack of harmful pesticides. Organic means more than "pesticide free"; it also means that the soil used to grow the vegetables meets requirements pertaining to mineral richness—much more so than conventional vegetables. Over time, mass-production processes have stripped the land of its minerals.

Some conventional vegetables and fruits, such as avocados and bananas, have such thick skins that the risk of contamination by pesticides is minimal. Others, such as berries and peppers, are particularly risky, so make a special effort to purchase those in organic form. If you must eat conventional vegetables, you can always ferment them to reduce the effects of pesticides.

You may notice that nutrient-dense, organically grown food tastes better; and because it provides you with more nourishment, you may need less of it to feel satisfied—thus effortlessly practicing calorie restriction!

I also recommend that you support your state CSA (community-supported agriculture) program and local farmers' markets, as they promote land stewardship and nonchemical production processes, and also build economically sustainable communities. At a time when one company, Monsanto, owns the entire world's supply of seeds, it is vital that we empower our local farmers and take back control of our food supply from corporate food giants.

No GMO . . . a Call to All

Another benefit of organic foods is that they are not genetically modified. Genetic modification alters the DNA of living organisms intended for human or animal consumption. The goal of gene-altered foods is to make them resistant to herbicides or to improve their nutritional value; however, they have been shown to have adverse effects on health and the environment.

It's important to note that we've been engineering plants for nearly 10,000 years through crossbreeding and cross-pollinating. Historically crop production has been successful because it follows classical breeding practices, which cross close relatives. With new GMO technologies, however, classical breeding is bypassed, so genetic information is crossed from one species to another to create an entirely different species. When you do this, you disrupt the complex ecosystem in which an organism lives and grows, impacting many forms of life, including bacteria and microbes.

In our immediate-gratification world, we want things bigger, juicier, sweeter, and prettier. If we can create a plant that is resistant to disease, then let's do it, we say, without any care for the long-term consequences.

The fact is, plants are *supposed* to become diseased. They are supposed to be attacked by pests and affected by seasonal and climate changes. This is a natural cycle, with some plants surviving and others not. The death of one organism sustains the life of another. This cycle may not always be pretty, but it is balanced and extremely precious.

We really don't know what might occur when we tamper with this process.

Seventy to eighty percent of all processed foods contain, or stem from, GMOs. Most Americans are not aware of the potential allergic or toxic reactions they may experience due to these genetically altered organisms. Because of poor labeling and scarcity of data, we may not see the threat of an allergic reaction until it has already hit us. For example, after genetically modified soy was introduced in the U.K., soy allergies skyrocketed 50 percent. Europe no longer allows genetically modified products, and some have suggested that Americans are being used as guinea pigs in a poorly regulated and untested industry.[7]

While it may be difficult to tell whether conventional vegetables are genetically modified, you can watch out for crops that typically are, such as soy, corn, cottonseed, canola, zucchini, Hawaiian papaya, and yellow squash. But there are many more that are being targeted. Go to **truefoodnow.org** for a list of brands of foods that are genetically engineered.

A Word on Fruit

Although the new USDA food plate, called "My Plate," has given almost equal priority to fruits and vegetables, Body Ecology recommends that you *favor land and ocean vegetables in your diet,* and give fruit less emphasis.

Certain fruits are healthy and provide a natural sweet taste that our bodies love. This is especially useful if we want to move from being too contracted—as we are when we first awaken in the morning—into a more balanced state. Fruits are expansive and help balance this dehydrated/contractive condition and therefore are best eaten in the morning on an empty stomach.

But fruit, if it is too sweet, weakens the adrenals—not good when you need energy to start your day. In fact, your adrenals need a boost of energy in the morning to get you up and going. The very sour juices listed in Chapter 12 are wonderfully energizing morning beverages. To make a really great, youthening "energy tonic," simply combine 1 ounce of a sour superfruit juice concentrate (like açaí or pomegranate) with 3–4 ounces of Body Ecology's probiotic liquids such as InnergyBiotic, Dong Quai, or CocoBiotic. Fruits have an alkalizing effect on the body when metabolized and are usually very good for us, but if your diet is high in sugar or if you feel as if your health, immunity, or energy levels are less than ideal, sweet fruit is harmful. While the sugar is "natural," it feeds opportunistic yeast and parasites, and, as mentioned previously, it can be especially weakening to your adrenals, particularly in the morning.

If your health, immunity, and energy levels are strong and you want to eat fruit, do so following the rules for food combining. This will ensure that you can enjoy it and digest it well without setting your body up for an inner-ecosystem imbalance. Fruits are cooling and hydrating, so as you follow the protocol, consider adding more during the summer when they are naturally in season.

The chart to follow shows the suggested fruits to include in your diet. Remember, the sour varieties have many health benefits and do not feed opportunistic yeast and parasites. If you are experiencing low energy levels or immune-related illness, only eat sour fruits. **Whenever you do eat fruit, always eat or drink something fermented.**

Fruit	Uses and Benefits
Lemon	Stimulates peristaltic action in your colon—try a glass of water with fresh-squeezed lemon and stevia (BED lemonade) to start your morning. Aids in digestion of protein. Has antiseptic properties and cleanses your digestive tract.
Lime	Same benefits as lemons.
Black-currant juice (unsweetened)	Soothes upset stomach and stimulates appetite. Great for anemia, high in vitamin C, and rich in antioxidants. Stimulates peristaltic action in your colon (try a glass of CocoBiotic with unsweetened black-currant juice and stevia to taste first thing in the morning). Strengthens the bladder and alleviates urinary tract infections. Excellent for the adrenals, the organs that provide energy.
Cranberry juice (unsweetened)	Strengthens the bladder and alleviates urinary tract infections (try 1 ounce of unsweetened cranberry-juice concentrate in 4 ounces of InnergyBiotic). Compounds in cranberry juice prevent pathogenic bacteria from adhering to the walls of your bladder.
Grapefruit	Low in sugar and has enough acidic qualities that it doesn't feed opportunistic yeast and parasites. The juice made from sour grapefruit is also beneficial.
Kiwi	Low in sugar and doesn't feed opportunistic yeast and parasites.
Berries— blueberries, raspberries, strawberries, bing cherries, and black- berries	Contain vitamins, minerals, and phytochemicals that may prevent disease. Dark-colored berries are high in antioxidants, which can help slow the aging process.

Sour green apples— Granny Smith	Fermenting green apples with your cultured veggies is a great idea because the microbiota will use the natural sugars in the apple for food. Also, when you make a green smoothie, a sour green apple adds a touch of sweetness but not too much. It's a much better choice than carrots, beets, or fennel.
Açaí	Packed with antioxidants that support healthy skin, hair, and nails.
Pomegranate	Has anti-inflammatory properties, helping protect you from cancer, cardiovascular disease, and harmful free radicals.
Noni juice	Aids proper digestion by stimulating bile flow and salivation. Promotes microbial balance in the gut. Healthy pH level supports immune function and inflammatory responses.
Sea buckthorn	Contains vitamins A, B_1, B_2, K, and E, and ten times the vitamin C of oranges, along with other antioxidants. The vivid orange to red pigmentation of sea buckthorn is attributed to high levels of carotenoids, which promote eye health.

As you move toward whole foods; add some new ones, such as sea vegetables and fermented veggies, to your diet; and reduce your sugar intake, you will be amazed by the youth and vitality you will gain. And you may be surprised to find that after a few weeks of adopting different eating habits, you start to crave vegetables. Your body, as it comes into balance with its newfound energy, will begin to signal you for the foods it needs, and some may be completely foreign to your palate.

The next chapter explores Body Ecology's grain-like seeds, a unique food and a pleasant answer to those universal carb cravings.

CHAPTER 11

GRAIN-LIKE SEEDS:
For Energy, Hydration, and Balance

Thousands of years old and venerated by those who grew them,
grain-like seeds have the power to make us turn back time.

When I was growing up, Wonder Bread was the coolest food around—the bread of choice for sandwiches. If you cut off the crust, you could roll it up into a gummy white ball. And its white wrapper, dotted with big yellow, blue, and red circles, made it seem even more fun. Little did any of us know we might as well have been eating glue.

Sixty-five percent of Americans eat a diet high in starchy carbs (mostly pasta, bread, and rice); and many of us often start our day with breakfast cereal, a slice of toast, or a doughnut. The recently popular high-protein diets have sought to address the obesity and diabetes issue in America by creating a new mind-set that all carbohydrates are "bad" and must be avoided. But just as with fats, this has created a lopsided picture and a heated health controversy. But just as it's the *type* of fat that's important, so the type of carbohydrate makes all the difference.

Not all carbohydrates are created equal. Table sugar, fruit, milk, grains, and vegetables are often lumped together into the category called "carbs" because they are made from or contain sugar. At Body Ecology, we disagree with classifying these foods as the same, and feel that it adds further confusion concerning what we should and should not eat.

We also make a clear distinction between refined sugars, grains and their flours, and grain-like seeds and *their* flours.

Finally, we believe vegetables should not be classified as carbs, but put into their own unique category. They are simply not "read" by the body in the same way as carbs. And there is such a wide variety enjoyed by humans—and so many to choose among each day—that they deserve their own category.

Empty, Refined Grains vs. Ancient, Whole Grain-like Seeds

To simplify the carb issue, we differentiate between "empty, re-fined grains," grains, and grain-like seeds. The first category—which includes bread, pasta, and cereals—should carry the skull-and-cross-bones label. They are nonnutritious, poisonous, aging, acid-forming foods. With such a label our mothers would have thought twice about giving us that slice of Wonder Bread!

The category that we would call "grains" would include wheat berries, oat groats, rice (there are many varieties), rye berries, barley, spelt, and so forth. This category may be beneficial for some people *if* the grains are prepared properly. They would be eaten in their whole form, soaked first to remove their enzyme inhibitors, and cooked slowly to make them more digestible. The problem with these grains, even if they are eaten in their whole form, is that they do contain a significant amount of sugar . . . potentially leading to acidity, infec-tions, inflammation, and earlier aging.

A third category, called "grain-like seeds," would include seeds that have many of the characteristics of grains. They are higher in protein yet lower in sugar than traditional grains, so they do not feed yeast or create inflammation in your body. Another added benefit is that they do not contain the protein *gluten,* which is present in grains such as wheat, spelt, rye, barley, and oats. Today, many of us are gluten intolerant, or if we have a genetic disorder called celiac sprue, we react severely to this protein. These grain-like seeds would still provide us with much-needed fiber and would help us remain calm and centered in the way that whole grains can do. When we eat them for our last meal of the day, they create serotonin, which turns into melatonin, which helps us sleep better at night.

Benefits of Body Ecology Grain-like Seeds

Grain-like seeds contain *phytoestrogens,* which help protect against harmful environmental and steroidal estrogens *(xenoestrogens)* that can get into your body through the food you eat, polluted air or water, or occupational exposure to chemical labs or industrial plants. Once in your body, they can stay in your tissues for years, causing hormone disruptions. Eating grain-like seeds can help balance hormones, support your immune system, and prevent or ease symptoms of osteoporosis and menopause. One important thing to keep in mind, however, is that *absorbing phytoestrogens only occurs if you have a healthy gut*—or inner ecosystem—teeming with friendly bacteria.

High in Fiber and Hydrating

The high fiber content of grain-like seeds is great for your digestive health, feeding friendly bacteria in your colon. These seeds are close enough to grains that they usually stop cravings for the refined carbs and cereals we are accustomed to eating. Grain-like seeds hold moisture in your intestines and help with constipation, which is often created by a dehydrated colon. Bulk fiber encourages peristaltic action in your intestines, moving food through your digestive system. Fiber pushes against the walls of your intestines, and they push back. Think of fiber as a personal trainer for your gut!

Nutrient-Dense for Calorie Curbing

Grain-like seeds are very high in nutrients, so you don't need much to help satisfy your body's requirements for proteins, vitamins, and minerals. If you are also eating fermented foods, you obtain even more nutrients from your meal, allowing you to eat less, while being more satisfied.

Now, let's take a closer look at the four grain-like seeds featured in the Body Ecology program—*amaranth, buckwheat, millet,* and *quinoa.*

Ancient Grains

These four superfoods may not be familiar to you yet, but they are delicious and readily available in grocery stores such as Whole Foods and in most health- or organic-food stores. All are high in protein, gluten free, and with the exception of buckwheat, alkaline forming. They are considered some of the most nutritionally complete foods available, and each one has a fascinating story to tell.

Amaranth

Amaranth, also called "Chinese spinach," was nearly exterminated from the planet! Actually a seed from a broad-leaf plant, this ancient yellow seed was a dietary staple among pre-Columbian peoples. The Aztecs, who fermented it into beer and popped its seeds like popcorn, used it prevalently and diversely. It also had a darker history . . . mixed with honey and human blood, it was consumed during religious rituals. For this reason, it was considered evil and was destroyed and banned by early Christian missionaries. It continued to be grown in remote villages in Mexico and Peru, and fortunately for us, it survived.[1]

Amaranth has three times the calcium of milk, so it is an excellent preventive therapy and treatment for osteoporosis. In addition, because it provides all eight essential amino acids (protein) but does not contain fat and cholesterol, it slows down the absorption of glucose into the bloodstream, making it easier to burn fat and lose weight. Unlike other grain-like seeds, amaranth contains *lysine* and *methionine,* which are both essential amino acids that must be obtained from the diet since they cannot be made by our bodies. Lysine has antiviral properties and is essential in the crosslink formation that stabilizes collagen and elastin—so it helps create younger-looking skin. Methionine helps with the detoxification pathways by supplying the body with sulfur, and it helps the liver process fats.

Uses:

There are 60 species of amaranth in the world. Amaranth has a sweet, peppery taste. Because of its distinctive flavor, many people combine it with other grains and grain-like seeds. It can be cooked, used as baking flour, added to stews and soups as a thickener, or made into a hot breakfast cereal or pilaf.

How to prepare:

Always wash thoroughly with a strainer under running water for a few minutes. Or soak 1 cup of amaranth in a pan of water overnight. In the morning, drain the old water, and put 3 cups of water in a pan with the amaranth. Simmer for 20 minutes. Drain and pour into a bowl. Add stevia, Lakanto, vanilla, or cinnamon butter; or eat it plain.

Buckwheat

Buckwheat has been around in America since colonial times, and was particularly common in the northeastern and north-central areas of the country, where it was grown on many farms and used as livestock feed. Native to both Northern Europe and Asia, buckwheat was brought to the U.S. in the 17th century by Dutch farmers, who called it *boekweit,* which means "beech wheat." It is a hardy plant that can withstand extremes in temperature and poor soil conditions.

Rich in flavonoids such as rutin (a phytonutrient that acts as an antioxidant) and a good source of B vitamins and magnesium (useful for improving blood flow and relaxing blood vessels), buckwheat contains all eight essential amino acids. Diets that contain buckwheat have been linked to lowered risk of developing high cholesterol and high blood pressure. Buckwheat is also a valuable food for diabetics, as it lowers glucose levels.

Uses:

Buckwheat is not a cereal grain, as most people think, but rather a fruit seed, related to rhubarb and sorrel. It is high in oxalates, so it should be avoided if you are on the low-oxalate diet. The hulled buckwheat grains are called "groats," and they make a traditional porridge called kasha. Buckwheat is sold either roasted or unroasted.[2] Unroasted buckwheat has a strong, nutty flavor, which roasting seems to mellow. Buckwheat also makes a great baking flour, is used in crackers and breads, and is a welcome alternative for people with gluten allergies . . . it makes a delicious pancake and fortifying breakfast cereal.

How to prepare:

Soaking buckwheat for at least 8 hours before cooking is recommended. It should be washed and rinsed thoroughly using a strainer. Add 1 part buckwheat to 2 parts boiling (salted) water or vegetable or kombu broth. After the liquid has returned to a boil, turn down the heat, cover, and simmer for about 20 minutes.

Millet

Millet is one of the oldest foods known to humankind, and it is even mentioned in the Bible. First cultivated in China, millet has been used in very hot, dry countries for thousands of years. In India, millet flour is used to make thin, flat cakes called *roti;* and in Africa, it is made into bread, baby food, and a thin breakfast porridge called *uji.*[3] The U.S. has traditionally used millet as livestock feed and birdseed. We are still quite uninformed about this ancient seed's amazing health benefits for humans.

Cancer-Fighting Power of Grains on Par with Vegetables

Research conducted by Rui Hai Liu, M.D., and his colleagues at Cornell University reveals that whole grains and grain-like seeds such as quinoa and millet contain many powerful cancer-fighting phytonutrients. Until recently, this had gone unrecognized because research methods were flawed.

Researchers have long known the power of phytonutrients, but they've been looking at only the "free" forms of these substances, which include one large class known as *phenolics*—potent antioxidants—which dissolve quickly and are immediately absorbed into the bloodstream. They have overlooked the "bound" forms of phenolics, which are attached to the walls of plant cells and must be released by intestinal bacteria during digestion before they can be absorbed.

Dr. Liu and his colleagues measured the relative amounts of phenolics, and whether they were present in bound or free form, in common fruits and vegetables such as apples, red grapes, broccoli, and spinach. In free form, the percentage of phenolics was quite high in these foods, while in grains the free form was almost nonexistent. However, these researchers also discovered that 99 percent of the phenolics *were* present in grains, but in "bound" form.

Because previous researchers had been using the same process to measure antioxidants in grains as they did with fruits and vegetables, they have, according to Liu, *vastly underestimated the amount and activity of antioxidants in whole grains.*

These findings, reported at the American Institute for Cancer Research (AICR) International Research Conference on Food, Nutrition and Cancer, underscore the message that **a variety of foods should be eaten for optimal health.** Says Liu, "Different plant foods have different phytochemicals. These substances go to different organs, tissues and cells, where they perform different functions. What your body needs to ward off disease is this synergistic effect—this teamwork—that is produced by eating a wide variety of plant foods, including whole grains."[i]

[i]Rui Hai Liu, M.D., as quoted at the American Institute for Cancer Research (AICR) International Research Conference on Food, Nutrition and Cancer, found at *Hook Up with Health* website, "Amazing Finding: Supplements vs. Whole Food," July 31, 2006, **http://hookupwithhealth.wordpress.com/2006/07/31/amazing-finding-suppliments-vs-whole-food** (accessed 1/6/10).

Rich in phytochemicals and one of the least allergenic grains out there, millet is nearly 15 percent protein and contains high amounts of fiber; B-complex vitamins, including niacin, thiamin, and riboflavin; the essential amino acids methionine and lecithin; and some vitamin E. It is the only grain that won't lose its alkaline state after cooking.

It is particularly high in the minerals iron, magnesium, phosphorus, and potassium, which are beneficial for the heart and can help lower cholesterol. Magnesium can help reduce the effects of migraines. Phosphorus is of particular importance as we age. It is an essential component of lipid-containing structures such as cell membranes, and it is necessary for the metabolism of fats. In addition to its role in forming the mineral matrix of bone, phosphorus is an essential component of numerous other life-critical compounds, including *adenosine triphosphate,* or ATP—the molecule that creates, stores, and transports energy in the body.[4]

Uses:
Millet is related to sorghum, looks a lot like maize, and comes in four varieties, including "pearl," which has the largest seeds and is the kind most often consumed by humans. Millet has a mildly sweet, nutlike flavor. It can be prepared as a cooked cereal; and is used in casseroles, breads, soufflés, and stuffing. It is a grain that mixes well with herbs and other seasonings. It also makes a unique kind of couscous and produces flour that yields a thin, buttery crust.

How to prepare:
Rinse millet off and remove any stones or unhulled pieces. It is recommended that you soak or sprout it for 8 to 24 hours prior to preparing it. Cook millet as you would rice but with more water (3 cups water to 1 cup millet). However, if you soak it, you won't need as much water when you cook it. After soaking, try 1 cup millet to 2 or 2½ cups water. You determine how much water to use depending on how soft you like your grain.

Quinoa

Quinoa (pronounced keen-wah) is native to the Andes of Bolivia, Chile, and Peru. A major staple of the altiplano Indians, and later the Incas, this versatile "mother grain" was believed to have been brought from heaven by a sacred bird called the *kullku*. Grown at 10,000 to 20,000 feet above sea level, quinoa allowed the altiplano peoples to thrive in the harsh living conditions that exist at such altitudes. Because these natives believed quinoa was a gift from the gods and contained spiritually enhancing qualities, the ritual first planting of the season was a godlike act performed by the emperor. Considered a god himself, the emperor was responsible for a successful quinoa harvest. He sowed the first seeds of the season with his golden *taquiza,* a planting stick.[5]

During the European conquest of South America, quinoa was scorned by the Spanish colonists as "food for Indians" and even actively suppressed. Because it imparted so much energy and strength, growing it was forbidden, on pain of death. Instead, the Spaniards introduced rice, wheat, and barley. Fortunately, quinoa still grew wild in the higher altitudes, where it could be hidden from the Spaniards, and small amounts were consumed in secret. But its ban had an irrevocable impact on the Incan culture. The grain fell into obscurity for centuries.[6]

Related to the spinach family, quinoa has been called "vegetable caviar" because of its nutrient and mineral density. It is one of the *most complete foods in nature* because it contains amino acids, enzymes, vitamins and minerals, fiber, antioxidants, and phytonutrients. The Food and Agricultural Organization (FAO) has compared its nutritional quality to that of dried whole milk, and the protein quality and quantity in the quinoa seed is superior to those of more common cereal grains. It is higher in calcium, phosphorus, magnesium, potassium, iron, copper, manganese, and zinc than wheat, barley, or corn; and it is rich in calcium and vitamins B and E. It is higher in lysine than wheat or rice, and contains a balanced set of essential amino acids for humans.

Quinoa is also gluten free and considered easy to digest. People living in the Andes consider it an *endurance food*. It is given to pregnant mothers to strengthen them, and is also used for altitude sickness. If you have a milk allergy—or are avoiding dairy—you still need calcium, and quinoa is a great alternative.

Quinoa's high mineral content also makes it excellent for bone health. The minerals manganese and copper act as antioxidants in your body to get rid of dangerous cancer- and disease-causing substances, while magnesium helps relax your muscles and blood vessels and positively affects blood pressure. Quinoa may be helpful if you suffer from migraines, diabetes, or atherosclerosis. High in fiber, it is a wonderful way to improve elimination and tone the colon.

Uses:

Quinoa is especially easy to cook and can be enjoyed year-round because it is versatile and light. You can use it in warming winter soups or refreshing summer salads. Quinoa's nutty flavor and rice-like texture make it perfect for stir-fries, but it can also be made into breads and biscuits. When cooked, quinoa is light, fluffy, slightly crunchy, and subtly flavored. Quinoa cooks quickly, which makes it a great breakfast meal; and it can be enjoyed in its whole-grain form, or you can try quinoa flakes made into a hot cereal as a wonderful replacement for oatmeal!

How to prepare:

Make sure you rinse your quinoa, and then soak it for at least 8 hours. Cook 25 minutes . . . and it's ready to mix with a variety of ingredients to create diverse and delicious meals. Adding a little Body Ecology InnergyBiotic to the soaking water is recommended. The beneficial microbiota help soften the grains before cooking, making them even more digestible.

(*Note:* Some of the nutritional information on these grain-like seeds that is contained in this section was drawn from **www .whfoods.com**.)

For many wonderful recipes using these four grains, please refer to the Body Ecology website or *The Body Ecology Diet* book.

Preparing Grains

It is always recommended that you soak your grain-like seeds for 8 to 24 hours. Grains, beans, seeds, and nuts all have phytic acid, an enzyme inhibtor, in them. It makes these foods difficult to break down in your digestive system. Since most people have weak digestive systems, especially as they age, eating grains without soaking them will mean they will be poorly digested, leading to a toxic, rapidly aging body.

What about Flour Made from Grain-like Seeds?

While the *whole* grain-like seeds are much more nutritious and are better for your digestion, health-food stores often sell *flours* made of buckwheat, millet, quinoa, and amaranth. You can also purchase breads made from these grains. Just like any flour product, the flour from Body Ecology–recommended grain-like seeds is mucus-forming and lacks fiber, which can actually be drying to your colon. If you suffer from constipation, avoid flour products at least until your inner ecosystem is recolonized with friendly bacteria and your elimination is excellent.

If you feel you must eat flour products, here's a suggestion. To offset the negative side of flour (even that of grain-like seeds), make it a habit to consume these products with fermented foods. Add cultured veggies to a sandwich, for example.

Konjaku—a Noodle Alternative That Won't Pack on the Pounds!

While we at Body Ecology recommend avoiding wheat products, there are wonderful pasta noodles made from quinoa and buckwheat (100 percent soba noodles). Another great high-fiber alternative to pasta is *konjaku* noodles, which are made from yam flour from the *konnyaku imo* tuber. A staple in Japan, konjaku noodles (also called *shirataki*) are gluten and calorie free, low carb, and won't feed bad bacteria and yeast in your digestive tract. The fiber in konjaku is called *glucomannan,* and it can control blood sugar and cholesterol and even help with "waist management." This is because konjaku noodles expand to many times their original size, making you feel full on less. They are great with stir-fried vegetables and Body Ecology sauces. Since they absorb other flavors well, season them liberally with herbs and other seasonings.

Grain-like Seeds and the Principle of 80/20

A balanced meal containing grain-like seeds would include 80 percent vegetables (land and ocean) and 20 percent grains. Following this principle will go a long way toward creating a healthy digestive system, and it will take the guesswork out of deciding how much of anything you need to include in your diet.

Like any new habit, it takes practice to get used to planning your meals this way. What starts to happen, though, is quite wonderful—you begin to feel comfortable in your own skin again, with less gas and bloating; a healthy weight; and a youthful, glowing appearance.

CHAPTER 12

HYDRATION CHOICES:
For Rejuvenation and Timeless Beauty

All health—beauty, stamina, strength, and youthfulness—
is intimately tied to the body's hydration levels.

In ancient Greek mythology, ambrosia was a substance that granted immortality to anyone who consumed it. Although it was never quite clear what this liquid "nectar" might actually be, it was very cleansing and purifying to all those who drank it or bathed in it. Hera (Juno in Roman mythology) used ambrosia to "cleanse all dirt from her fair body,"[1] and it was believed to undo the cumulative toll of years. Its restorative attributes could turn back the hands of time.

There is really only one liquid on the planet that has the purifying reverse-the-clock qualities of ambrosia. It's water—literally, the elixir of the gods.

Approximately 60 to 70 percent of the body and 85 percent of the brain is composed of water—the universal solvent and the most abundant substance inside of us. Since the beginning of life within Earth's primordial ocean, we have essentially been water-based life-forms. And virtually all of our chemical and physical processes; nerve transmissions; and circulatory, motor, and immune functions occur in or depend on this water-based terrain.

But this is just the tip of the iceberg, so to speak. The work of Masaru Emoto has demonstrated water's unique trans-spiritual qualities as well, and its startling ability to be transformed by positive or negative energy.

A doctor of alternative medicine, Emoto gathered water samples from around the world, slowly froze them, and then photographed them with a dark-field microscope to capture their aesthetic and structural differences. Emoto discovered that there were radical discrepancies in the crystalline structures of water depending on its source and the surrounding environment. For example, water from a pure mountain spring might reveal a beautiful geometric design, while water taken from a polluted or heavily industrial area might show structures that appear random and distorted.

Noting how water changed in different environments and under different conditions, Emoto began to wonder if music, words, and even thoughts might also affect the crystal structures. He then conducted a number of experiments where he exposed water in glasses to different words, pictures, or music. He photographed these as well.[2]

The resulting images are truly astounding—Google Emoto's name and you'll find many examples. Once you've seen the shimmering jewel of *peace* versus the jagged-edged cavity of *anger,* you can't help but be convinced of the transformative impact that we have on water and that water has on us. If so much of who we are is made up of water, consider how important our own thoughts and intentions can be to our health and well-being.

Dehydration—What It Means and What It Does

We often hear of nutrients that are "good for" radiant skin and hair, or are "essential" to a strong heart or proper digestion. But most of us don't realize how much of our physical and mental well-being depends on being well hydrated.

You may be excited to learn that water can be a therapy; a healing substance for your body.

What does it actually mean to be *dehydrated?* Most people think of dehydration as simply the body lacking in water. But a more accurate discussion of dehydration would include looking at *where that water is located.*

Like fish in an aquarium, all of our cells are surrounded by a complex *modified* water called the extracellular fluid. When we become dehydrated, 66 percent of the water loss is from the *interior* of our cells (the intracellular fluid) and 26 percent is lost from the extracellular volume.[3] Dehydration causes the blood to become concentrated.

The mineral-rich extracellular fluid creates a kind of buffer zone against toxins. Some physiologists refer to this fluid *and* the complex network of fibrous connective proteins as the extracellular *matrix*—a distinct system within the body, even larger than your skin surface. According to the matrix theory, you are only as healthy as your matrix. It provides nutrition to your cells, removes waste, regulates your internal environment, "reads" your external environment, defends your cells against free radicals, and more.[4]

But when the *interiors* of cells become dehydrated, it is nothing short of a cellular nightmare. Acid builds up inside, the cells become poisoned, and DNA damage occurs. Enzymes and amino acids lose their effectiveness. Brain cells, lacking useful amino acids, cannot manufacture neurochemicals, such as serotonin. The electrical and magnetic energy inside each cell is lost, weakening its vitality. The list goes on and on.

The initial impact of *mild* dehydration in adults appears when the body has lost about 2 percent of its total fluid. Some of these mild dehydration effects[5] include:

- Thirst
- Loss of appetite
- Dry skin
- Flushing
- Dark-colored urine
- Dry mouth/cotton mouth
- Fatigue/weakness
- Chills
- Head rushes

However, when dehydration is long-term or "chronic," even if low-grade, the symptoms take on the additional characteristics of chronic degenerative diseases:

- Fatigue/energy loss
- Constipation
- Digestive disorders
- Feeling irritable
- Feeling depressed
- Not sleeping well
- Increased cravings for sugar and carbs
- Fear of crowds or of leaving the house
- Poor circulation and congestion of lymph glands
- High or low blood pressure
- Gastritis and stomach ulcers
- Respiratory troubles
- Acid/alkaline imbalance
- Excess weight/obesity
- Eczema
- Elevated cholesterol
- Cystitis and urinary infections
- Rheumatism
- Premature aging
- Skin aging, including wrinkles and loss of elasticity

In short, the health effects of chronic dehydration are profound.

F. Batmanghelidj was a renowned medical doctor who wrote extensively about water's healing properties for more than 22 years. His research revealed that the issue of dehydration is sorely misunderstood—even by medical doctors and by the alternative-health community.

Dr. B (as he was affectionately called) was not saying that you could heal diseases with water alone, but that if you want to stay young, and even reverse many of the signs and symptoms of aging and disease, you must address and correct your lifelong problem of not being well hydrated.

Drinking enough water to stay well hydrated is one of those issues that we understand *intellectually:* "Yes, I know I should be drinking more water, but . . ."

This can be a difficult habit to learn, as most of us didn't grow up watching our parents or grandparents drink water. The trend of carrying around bottled water is a very recent one, and many of us still do not understand water's profound importance.

Young bodies are blessed with optimal hydration. A baby's body is 80 percent water, while that of an adult is only 60 to 70 percent. As we age, this percentage continues to drop. To regain our youthfulness, we must be mindful to keep water nearby and make a conscious effort to achieve optimal hydration at all times.

The Amazing Benefits of Water

Batmanghelidj's first book, *Your Body's Many Cries for Water,* is a testament to the extensive health benefits that can be accomplished solely by restoring sufficient hydration levels. In this book he documented the many health conditions he was able to reverse with just ordinary water, minerals, and sea salt.

Most hydration cures are related to the fact that water is the primary transport system in our bodies. It carries nutrients and oxygen into the cells and waste products out. When hydration is not at an optimal level, blood turns acidic, so it thickens and becomes more condensed. As it does so, circulation decreases, and there is poor oxygenation of tissue and inefficient removal of CO_2 and toxins. All this creates a low-grade state of metabolic acidosis. Remember, when we're too acidic, our bodies become *dis*-eased.

When toxins and waste products accumulate in our cells, the cells then deteriorate or even die. As these tissue cells die, aging results.

Skin sags, hair falls out, energy drops, memory fails, hormone levels plummet, libido wanes, and heart attacks and aneurysms can occur. Further, dehydration prevents accumulations from being washed out of the cells and tissues. These accumulations, such as cholesterol, lactic-acid wastes, pyruvic crystals, or calcium, muck up the cell membranes, clog the efficient pathways of arteries, and inhibit the smooth motion of the joint capsules; and thus contribute to such chronic degenerative diseases as arteriosclerosis, arthritis, gout, kidney stones, and gallstones, to name a few.

Water is the substance that takes the toxins and carbon dioxide out and carries vital nutrients in. That is why it can and should be considered an anti-aging remedy!

Its benefits[6] are numerous:

- Water makes the skin smoother.

- Water helps reduce fatigue.

- Water makes the immune system function more efficiently.

- Water helps with weight management.

- Water helps prevent the loss of memory as we age; and reduces the risk of Alzheimer's, Parkinson's, and Lou Gehrig's disease.

- Water can help offset the progression and symptoms of hormone-related health issues such as hot flashes and osteoporosis.

- Water is the main lubricant in the joint spaces and helps prevent arthritis.

- Water rids the body of toxins.

Batmanghelidj also showed that dehydration causes your body to produce excessive amounts of cholesterol. Why would this be so?

Batmanghelidj called cholesterol a "waterproof bandage." When blood becomes dehydrated and therefore too concentrated and imbalanced, it rushes through our arteries and capillaries, creating abrasions and tears. Cholesterol is produced to cover them up. If this "bandage" were not there, then blood would get under the arterial membrane and peel it off, soon killing us.[7]

How Do We Get Dehydrated in the First Place?

Through activities of daily living, the average person loses about three to four liters (about 10 to 15 cups) of fluid a day in sweat, urine, exhaled air, and bowel movement. We lose approximately one to two liters of water just from breathing. The most common cause of increased water loss is exercise and sweating. The evaporation of sweat from the skin accounts for 90 percent of our cooling ability.

Exercise, sweating, diarrhea, temperature, or altitude can significantly increase the amount of water we lose each day. Even though we are all at risk of dehydration, the people most vulnerable are infants, elderly adults, and athletes. They are not able either to adequately express their thirst sensation or to detect it and do something in time.

What we lose must be replaced by the fluids we drink and the food we eat.

Tips for Staying Hydrated

Staying properly hydrated is one of the best—and easiest-to-implement—anti-aging strategies around, but it is one we must be vigilant about.

- It's important to drink regularly, not just when you "feel" thirsty. Most likely, as you grow older, your thirst sensation will completely disappear, and you will not be able to recognize that your body is dehydrated. In other words, don't depend on the symptom of a "dry mouth" to alert you to the need to drink water again. Keep a glass or bottle beside you at all times.

- To keep your body well hydrated, drink at least half your body weight in ounces. If you weigh 200 pounds, drink ten or more 12-ounce glasses of water per day. If you weigh 100 pounds, you need at least four or more 12-ounce glasses per day. If you are physically active or live in a warm climate, drink even more.

- A hydrated body produces clear, colorless urine every three to four hours. If your urine is yellow, you are dehydrated—but only moderately so. If your urine is orange or dark colored, you are severely dehydrated.

- If your water-drinking habits are poor, try this tip: Set a timer for 60 minutes. Every time it goes off, drink one cup of water. Set the timer again. If you don't like the idea of using a timer, another suggestion is to keep a running list of what you drink each day on a notepad at your work desk or perhaps on your refrigerator at home. That way you can see when you are falling behind. If necessary, place sticky notes everywhere that remind you to pour a delicious, life-lengthening glass of water.

- When you wake up in the morning, *immediately* drink two glasses of water to rehydrate after loss of fluids during the night. You wake up dehydrated, toxic, and in need of energy to start the day. It's best to then wait at least 30 minutes before consuming other foods. Water early in the morning gets your circulation going and herds those toxins out of the body.

- To keep your body and brain functioning at peak performance, consider having at least half your daily water intake before noon . . . it really revitalizes a dehydrated body.

- Drink two glasses of water 30 minutes before lunch and again before dinner. This will help your digestive tract (and liver) do a better job of processing the food you eat.

- Do not drink water with meals. Large amounts taken with a meal will dilute stomach acid. Instead, try chewing each mouthful of food at least 30 to 40 times before swallowing.

- Wait about one hour after each meal and drink another glass of water.

- Sipping on a warm cup of tea with meals has a positive effect on digestion. While warm liquids (including soup) with a meal can aid digestion, ice-cold drinks halt it and, in general, are a shock to your system. You can also sip on three to four ounces of one of Body Ecology's probiotic liquids, such as CocoBiotic. Served in a pretty champagne glass, it is a superior substitute for wine.

- Dr. B taught that water combined with other ingredients has an "agenda" and cannot be counted as part of your daily water intake. However, minerals and sea salt can be added. The more water you drink, the more salt you need. The ocean and your blood are nearly identical in the proportion of mineral electrolytes.

- Forget the coffee break. Take water breaks instead. Water is the source of true energy, and coffee is dehydrating.

- If you find it difficult to up your daily amount of water, it is strongly suggested that you read Dr. F. Batmanghelidj's book *Water for Health, for Healing, for Life: You're Not Sick, You're Thirsty!* This is an update to *Your Body's Many Cries for Water.* It will definitely convince you to drink more water.

The Search for Pure Water

The best water in the world—the ambrosia of those early Greeks—is found very deep in the earth, about two miles down. It is called "primal water," and it is water that has been untouched by the atmosphere. It surfaces through fissures in rocks. Unfortunately, this water is largely unavailable to us and quite costly. Scientists also fear that even it may contain some undesirable constituents such as metals, radioactivity, and even hydrocarbons.

Sadly, healthy water is not available anymore from our city water systems. Water-treatment chemicals and additives (for example, chlorine, chloramines, aluminum, and fluoride); microorganisms; pollution; heavy metals; and even medicinal drugs such as antidepressants and antibiotics that cannot be filtered out (from human and animal urine) have compromised our drinking and bathing water, perhaps forever.

These contaminants have caused people from developed countries—including half of all Americans—to turn to bottled water as their primary source of drinking water. The bottled-water craze, which began in the 1990s, has grown steadily to a $100-billion-a-year industry. The results are predictably negative:

- It's expensive. At up to $2.50 per liter ($10 per gallon), bottled water costs more than gasoline in the United States.

- A lot more energy and raw materials are required to produce and transport bottled water compared to tap water. Worldwide, some 2.7 million tons of plastic are used to bottle water each year.

- Most plastic bottles are not recycled, and end up in the ocean or in a landfill.

- Even though the very best bottled waters may start out chemically and biologically pure, plastic bottles may pose some risks, as they can leach chemicals into the water itself, especially if they have been sitting in the hot sun.

What You Can Do

Make your first priority the installation of a water-filtration system in your home. You should be aware that roughly 40 percent of bottled water starts as tap water, so simply switching from tap to bottles is not the best answer.

Why not go green, especially if you are traveling away from home? Carry a *refillable, protected* glass water bottle or an HDPE (#2 high-density polyethylene) plastic bottle, preferably made by a trusted supplier (such as Nalgene). Never choose a plastic bottle (#7 Lexan or polycarbonate), which can leach BPA, a toxin, into the water. *Note:* At Body Ecology we do not recommend stainless-steel bottles because most are manufactured in China and can leach metals (including troublesome nickel) into the pure water.

At home, the very best way to keep water pure is in a refillable glass bottle.

Distilled Water

Distilled water is water that has been boiled and evaporated. The vapor (or steam) leaves the impurities behind, then cools and condenses back to pure water. This is the process nature uses to recycle water on planet Earth. Water evaporates from the oceans, and the wind currents carry it over cooler mountainous areas, where it condenses into rain and snow. This process eradicates virtually all microbiological impurities—including protozoa, bacteria, and viruses—and heavy metals. It contains no minerals, so it is able to actively absorb toxic substances and eliminate them from the body quickly.

Distilled water has long been popular among people who embark upon a fast or detoxification regimen, although the benefits and risks have been the subject of debate for many decades. The problem, some opponents argue, is that distilled water is so "pure" and chemically "hungry" that it will dissolve minerals out of the body. Proponents of distilled water argue that the amount of minerals supplied by water is insignificant compared to dietary minerals, so this is a moot point. They claim that the benefit of extracting toxins from the body's tissues outweighs any negative aspects. Yet another perspective is that as soon as distilled water mixes with the stomach fluids, it quickly loses much of its chemical "hunger" and is no different from other low-mineral sources.

You should be cautious about using distilled water (or any low-mineral-content water) during fasting, especially if you are deficient in minerals already, as you might experience heart irregularities and a rise in blood pressure. If you are eating a healthy diet or supplementing the distilled water with a mineral mixture, this should balance the potential removal of minerals.

Those toxic soft drinks and colas that so many uninformed Americans consume are made with low-mineral-content water. Added to this are acidic ingredients such as phosphoric acid and high-fructose corn syrup. This combination results in the loss of significant amounts of calcium, magnesium, and other trace minerals. The more mineral loss, the greater the risk for osteoporosis, osteoarthritis, hypothyroidism, coronary artery disease, high blood pressure, and a long list of degenerative diseases associated with premature aging.

Generally, the consumption of distilled water as a means of hydration should be limited unless an adequate diet and complete mineral supplementation are in place.

A Water Process You Can Live With:
Reverse Osmosis + Coconut-Shell Activated Carbon

At Body Ecology, we recommend a water filter that uses both reverse osmosis and coconut-shell activated carbon. This tank-less system is the most effective, practical, and economical for making the highest-quality, contaminant-free water for drinking and cooking. If you use ice, make sure you are using this pure, high-quality water to make it. And, of course, you'll want to also give it to your pets. Information on this water filter can be obtained at: **www.bodyecology.com**.

Sparkling Water vs. Still Water—
Some "Fizzy" Misconceptions

Although sparkling waters are consumed all over the world, most people aren't aware that they vary widely in taste, quality, purity, and origin. It is important when choosing "fizzy" over "flat" that you select only those that are naturally carbonated. What does "naturally carbonated" mean? Certain geological conditions can produce naturally carbonated water, such as volcanic activity. When water comes in contact with certain geological formations, it takes on a strong and healthy mineral composition, which the carbon dioxide in the water helps absorb. Some waters may have been formed only 30 days before bottling, whereas others are more than 20,000 years old. It's the mineral content that really makes these waters uniquely curative.

Ideal for the human body is alkaline water, which contains minerals such as calcium, silica, and magnesium. This is why sparkling water may be a better option than still, and is certainly better than distilled, which has no "life force" energy.

There is a long-standing belief that sparkling water is not as healthy as springwater, but new research indicates otherwise.

A study published in *The Journal of Nutrition* was designed to assess the difference in health benefits between women who drank sparkling mineral water and women who drank still mineral water. Study participants were asked to drink one liter of either the sparkling or still water each day for two months, followed by two months on the other water. During the study, the participants underwent a number of tests, including blood pressure and cholesterol levels.

Compared to the still mineral water, the drinking of sparkling water brought about significant reductions in the level of LDL cholesterol (generally regarded as a risk factor for heart disease), as well as a significant increase in levels of HDL cholesterol (generally taken to reduce heart-disease risk). These and other biochemical changes induced by drinking sparkling water were estimated to reduce the women's risk of developing heart disease over the next decade by about one-third.[8]

Researchers aren't completely sure why sparkling water is good for so many of us, but they suspect it has something to do with the high mineral content in naturally carbonated water and its ability to stimulate bicarbonate (HCO_3) secretion in both the stomach and the duodenum. (Remember, though, this is not necessarily true for all carbonated waters such as those with little mineral content or the wrong kind.) Although such waters are often high in sodium—a mineral that has often been maligned and erroneously linked to high blood pressure and heart problems—it is believed that the bicarbonate alkalinity and the other minerals in sparkling water help balance any negative effects sodium may have in the body.

Minerals also determine differences in taste. As with wine, subtle flavor distinctions can be caused by the soil, climate, and geography of where the water is "harvested." The amount of mineral elements in water is commonly referred to as "total dissolved solids" (TDS) and is expressed in milligrams per liter (mg/l) or parts per million (ppm). TDS is made up of positively charged cations (sodium, calcium, magnesium, potassium, phosphorus, iron, manganese, copper, and strontium) and negatively charged anions (chloride, bicarbonate, carbonate, sulfate, fluoride, and silicate)—and many trace elements. Altogether, there are about 80 mineral-element building blocks. The higher the mineral content, the more distinctive the taste. You might think of low TDS as comparable to white wine, with more of a neutral taste that's less weighty. Waters with high TDS feel heavier and have more of an aftertaste, rather like a robust red wine. In the U.S., bottled water must contain at least 250 mg/l TDS in order to qualify as "mineral" water.[9]

Other studies have suggested that the magnesium and bicarbonate content of natural mineral water can result in favorable changes in urinary pH and magnesium and citrate excretion, and may inhibit kidney-stone formation (from oxalates).[10]

But not all sparkling waters are what they seem (or what they're promoted to be). For example, many people consider Perrier the "aristocracy" of carbonated waters, but the truth is that Perrier (475 mg/l TDS) is a still water that has been aggressively infused with CO_2 bubbles, creating unusual acidity (pH of 5.5).

Instead of Perrier, drink Apollinaris (1,600 mg/l TDS) or a water from Germany called Gerolsteiner (2,527 mg/l TDS). Gerolsteiner is almost like taking a mineral supplement. Classified as naturally carbonated, with a low pH, this water has been a famous health tonic since 1888. (It is interesting to note that the TDS of these waters is so high that they exceed the maximum allowed for drinking water in the U.S.)

For more information on where to purchase the finest waters and to find out which ones are the healthiest, go to: **www.aquamaestro .com/step1.asp**.

For additional information on various waters, go to: **www.fine waters.com.** Or read the book *Fine Waters: A Connoisseur's Guide to the World's Most Distinctive Bottled Waters,* by Michael Mascha, which can be purchased at: **www.finewaters.com/Bottled_Water_Guide_ Book.asp**.

The Important Role of Salt and Minerals

As you increase the amount of water you drink, you should also increase your intake of mineral-rich sea salt and other minerals.

Body Ecology's Ancient Earth Minerals is an excellent choice for minerals from a *land* source, while Celtic sea salt is the recommended way to obtain minerals from the *ocean.* Ideally, you want both. In the next chapter we'll discuss more about what makes an ideal sea salt, and where to get it.

Don't be afraid of salt . . . not if it is high-quality, mineral-rich sea salt. Salt is not bad for you. It does not raise blood pressure if you also have adequate amounts of other minerals, especially potassium, calcium, magnesium, and zinc, in your diet. These key minerals work with sodium to keep the right balance of water inside and outside the cells (osmotic balance).

If you want to begin reversing the signs and symptoms of aging, balance your sodium intake with your water consumption—drink more water, yes, but also consume sea salt and minerals. Dr. Bat-manghelidj's many years of research clearly showed this. His recommendation is to take a quarter teaspoon of sea salt per *quart* of water—that's every four to five glasses of water. This helps increase aldosterone, an important hormone made in our adrenals.

Three capsules of Ancient Earth Minerals can be taken in the morning with your water and a quarter teaspoon of sea salt. Repeat this again at bedtime.

Other Hydration Choices

A dangerous misconception has many of us thinking that other fluids such as coffee, tea, soda, wine, alcoholic beverages, juices, and milk count toward our daily water requirements. Dr. Batmanghelidj made it very clear that these other fluids have their own "agenda." This means they contain chemicals that alter the body's chemistry at its central-nervous-system control centers. Even milk differs from water—it should be considered a food, not a substitute for water.[11]

Your body was designed to drink pure water that has no agenda. Although other healthy hydration choices appear in the pages to follow, please remember that none should take the place of the right amount of pure water your unique body needs each day. *Nothing is a substitute for water!*

Super Green Drinks

You may be familiar with a variety of supernutrient green drinks sold in powder form that are widely available in health-food stores today. These drinks are quite popular, and rightly so. Typically, a blend of powerful, energizing, whole foods and herbs, in a base of cereal grasses and microalgae, is stirred into water or juice. Green drinks are easy to digest and provide an excellent all-alkaline option first thing in the morning. This will help bring your body, which becomes more acidic at night, back into balance. Green drinks are a great way to help correct nutritional deficiencies—you get so many amazing nutrients in one drink—and they are much better than taking supplements.

Look for a green drink that has healing benefits of aiding digestion; creating energy; and providing protein, enzymes, vitamins, minerals, and probiotics. Many green drinks have spirulina, collards, and kale, which in raw form can suppress the thyroid. But this is not so when they are fermented! A well-blended formula can be such an excellent energizer in the morning that you might find that it replaces your need for caffeine. A whole-food green drink also works well if you are having a midafternoon slump and need a pick-me-up.

Body Ecology's green drink, Vitality SuperGreen, does all of the above. Super Spirulina Plus is another excellent protein powder. One hundred percent of its ingredients are fermented. Over 50 percent of this is predigested, fermented spirulina. Google the many extraordinary benefits of spirulina and see why we at Body Ecology are so excited to bring this superfood to the marketplace in a fermented form. Fermentation increases the bioavailability hundreds of times over.

Tea

Tea has many healing qualities, including polyphenols and tannins. Polyphenols in tea provide antioxidants, increase white blood cells, and may have anticancer properties. They also absorb cholesterol in the digestive tract and bloodstream. Tannins and oils in tea can aid digestion and fat emulsification. All foods have a positive and a negative. Black and green tea are high in oxalates.

Green teas vary in taste because of differences in soils, harvesting, and processing. Green tea is not processed as heavily as other teas because the freshly picked leaves are dried and then heat-treated to prevent oxidation. With the finer varieties, traditional handmade methods are often used; and the resulting tastes can range from sweet, buttery, nutty, and smoky to grassy and floral.

More and more research substantiates the health benefits stemming from regular consumption of green tea. Specifically, it contains a group of antioxidants known as *catechins,* which protect our cells from free radicals. They can actually prevent tumor-generating conditions that can lead to cancer. Catechins may also prove beneficial for the treatment of existing cancer and the prevention of heart disease.[12]

Research has also shown that green tea increases your metabolism, acts as an antiviral, inhibits oral bacterial plaque, is a rich source of vitamins, and has anti-aging properties. It, as well as ginger tea, is an excellent digestive aid. There are several other teas with medicinal properties, too. Cat's claw, echinacea, and pau d'arco (also known as Brazilian bark or taheebo) are especially healing and antifungal. Burdock-root teas, dandelion-root teas, and the Yogi brand blend

"Stomach Ease" are also quite healing. Fruit teas and teas with citric acid are best avoided, as they often have mold growing on them. Teas such as tulsi (also known as holy basil) and chamomile are calming and can help manage stress and regulate sleep.

Consider using teas as a means of warmth and comfort, consumed in addition to your daily water requirements, but not in place of water. As mentioned previously, having a cup of warm tea or a bowl of soup adds liquid to your meals, and helps facilitate the digestive process. Tea can also be your between-meals snack, providing warming, healthy liquid—and even a touch of sweetness—to satisfy a craving. If you like your teas a little sweet, be sure to use stevia instead of processed sugar or artificial sweeteners.

You can find many green teas in grocery stores today, but there is often a big difference in quality, purity, and taste. If you fancy yourself a tea connoisseur, then you will certainly enjoy the rare and unusual varieties offered by artisan tea makers. One example is Silk Road Teas (**www.silkroadteas.com**).

Unlike most tea companies, Silk Road buys its teas direct, and is always searching for new regions that produce unique-tasting varieties. They sell only 100 percent unadulterated leaf. Their teas are certified organic, too, which means they are grown without the use of chemicals and pesticides, with no added flavorings, colorings, perfumes, oils, or preservatives. With a mission to support the artisan or traditional tea farms in China, Silk Road delivers teas that have a nuanced, healthful taste; and that are now widely recognized for their unparalleled quality and purity.

Wine

Many readers will be very disappointed to learn that wine is not the anti-aging beverage that the media has led us to believe. It's true that red wine has *resveratrol,* the anti-aging substance that mimics calorie restriction. But wine is also, like all alcohol, very dehydrating.

Dr. Batmanghelidj's research clearly showed that alcohol stops the emergency water-supply system to important cells, such as the ones in your brain.

Wine is fermented, yes, but it is fermented from fruit and contains *wild* yeast. When your immune system is already fighting a battle to bring a systemic yeast infection under control, wild fermentation (used in beer, alcohol, and kombucha) is not good for anyone with candidiasis. Wine does contain resveratrol, but wine is not a *healing* drink, as are the other fermented foods and liquids mentioned throughout the book. If you are really serious about reversing the signs of aging in your body, avoid wine. If you feel you must drink it, limit it to special occasions and celebrations, and be sure to take in even more water as soon as possible, especially water with minerals and a quarter teaspoon of Celtic sea salt. A meal with a glass of wine *and* a serving of cultured vegetables will help balance the negative side effects of the alcohol.

While many of us are accustomed to learning about and enjoying different types of wines—finding out about the regions they come from and discovering the subtleties of taste and how well they pair with certain foods—we can also bring the same enthusiasm to tea. There are so many varieties, each with its own unique properties that benefit the body in some specialized way. Consider experimenting with tea with the same zest you bring to your wine tasting!

CocoBiotic: A Naturally Fermented, Refreshing Probiotic Drink Made from Young Coconuts

All probiotics are not the same! Many probiotic products are synthesized in a laboratory . . . even worse, many of them are genetically modified.

Not CocoBiotic.

A naturally fermented drink created from wild-crafted young Thai coconut, CocoBiotic utilizes Grainfield's proprietary *FermFlora* organic fermentation process. The gut-friendly bacteria and yeasts in this delicious beverage are derived entirely from nature . . . from organically certified plant sources.

With a light, refreshing, and slightly fizzy taste, this beverage has long been a favorite of Body Ecology customers. While CocoBiotic is *not* exactly the same thing as young coconut kefir, and not made in the same way, it *does* similarly embrace Body Ecology's emphasis on fermentation, and provides you with an amazing range of health benefits. Fermented young coconut juice was included *by design* . . . because of the many benefits coconut-kefir users have reported over the years, such as:

- Improved digestion
- Reduced sugar cravings
- Greatly increased energy
- Improved cleansing of the liver

Healthy Celebrations:
Now That's *Really* Something to Toast!

Instead of wine or bubbly, pour InnergyBiotic or CocoBiotic into that pretty champagne glass. It lends a little elegance to your meals and aids in digestion. It is also a great way to celebrate a special occasion because you can drink it knowing you are going to live a long and healthy life.

Juices from the Sour-Fruit Family

There are many *unsweetened* fruit-juice concentrates that can be used to make excellent energy-boosting juices in the morning. Look for cranberry, black-currant, pomegranate, açaí, noni, mangosteen, and blueberry *concentrates.*

Read the labels carefully and purchase them only if they are unsweetened.

Unfortunately, many manufacturers and marketers of these juices add water, additional fruit juices and concentrates, sweeteners, chemical preservatives, and other unwanted and unnecessary ingredients. This is done to lower costs, improve flavor, increase sweetness, and speed production runs.

The sour juices mentioned in the following pages are gaining in popularity and are often called "superfruits." Consider adding them to water, young coconut kefir, or milk kefir for a delicious, hydrating drink first thing in the morning. Use stevia or Lakanto to turn them from sour to deliciously sweet.

— **Noni:** Traditionally an important fermented food for those living in the Polynesian islands, noni is high in minerals; contains trace minerals; and has numerous health benefits, including helping increase production of serotonin, strengthening immunity, increasing microbial populations in the intestines, and regulating blood sugar and energy levels. Unfortunately, noni has to be pasteurized or it would continue to ferment during shipping, and the glass bottles would explode. Genesis Today is a recommended brand for noni juice.

— **Mangosteen:** The rind of this fruit from Thailand and Myanmar has been shown to have medicinal qualities. In Southeast Asia, it has been used to treat dysentery and skin disorders, such as eczema. Mangosteen is a free-radical scavenger. It supports healthy inflammatory processes, strengthens the immune system, and promotes youthful cell regeneration and thus, healthy aging. Genesis Today's mangosteen juice is 100 percent pure, is wild-harvested, and is made the traditional way, just like it was 1,000 years ago. Mangosteen is pasteurized, also.

— **Açaí:** A purple berry from Brazil, açaí falls into the category of "superfruit." It is thought to have anti-aging and anticancer benefits, along with promoting improved digestion, mental focus, and energy. More studies are being done to better understand the health benefits of açaí. Genesis Today also has premium-quality unsweetened açaí juice. Açaí is usually pasteurized, although if you find the pulp frozen, it may or may not be.

— **Pomegranate:** A fruit that grows wild in many parts of the world, pomegranates are rich in phytochemicals, and have been shown to inhibit hormone-dependent breast-cancer-cell growth. A report published in a recent issue of *The American Association for Cancer Research* reveals that compounds found in pomegranate have a suppressive effect on the proliferation of breast-cancer cells.[13] Pomegranate has also been shown to lower bad cholesterol and to reverse plaque buildup in the arteries.

— **Black currant:** This fruit is revered in Europe as an adrenal tonic to provide energy. It also helps soothe an upset stomach and stimulates appetite. It is great for anemia, is high in vitamin C and rich in antioxidants, and strengthens the bladder while helping to alleviate urinary tract infections. It also stimulates peristaltic action in your colon. Try a glass of water with unsweetened black-currant juice (and stevia to taste) first thing in the morning. The brand Austria's Finest, Naturally imports an excellent black-currant juice (**www .austrianpumpkinoil.com**).

— **Cranberry:** This berry strengthens the bladder and alleviates urinary tract infections. Research shows compounds in cranberry juice prevent pathogenic bacteria from adhering to bladder walls.

— **Blueberry:** This unassuming little berry packs a wallop—with possibly the highest antioxidant capacity of any fruit or vegetable because of its large concentration of anthocyanin (the pigment that gives it its free-radical-fighting powers and which is also an anti-inflammatory). Blueberries have been shown to slow down vision loss, improve brain functioning, and be anti-hypoglycemic. And recent studies point to this berry's benefits to diabetics due to its ability to improve fasting glucose and insulin sensitivity.

— **Lemons and limes:** Lemons and limes contain unique flavonoid compounds that have antioxidant and anticancer properties. They are also an excellent source of vitamin C, which is a powerful antioxidant that has been shown to be helpful in reducing some of the symptoms of arthritis. Vitamin C supports the immune system, and a little extra can be a great preventive first step when you feel a cold coming on. There are also compounds in citrus fruits—called *limonoids*—that have been shown to help fight cancers of the mouth, skin, lung, breast, stomach, and colon.

Additionally, lemon juice can help alleviate symptoms of indigestion—such as heartburn and bloating—and, in general, it helps your body to eliminate waste more efficiently, mitigating problems with constipation and diarrhea. Better yet, it stimulates the liver, helps dissolve uric acid and other poisons, and liquefies bile.

Sour fruits are wonderful, hydrating, nutritious, antioxidant-rich, and refreshing foods that can be part of your anti-aging arsenal. But be careful to follow your body's signals as you learn to develop a sense of when and if you need the expansive, cooling properties of fruits. Keep in mind the principles that allow your body to best assimilate them.

Dehydration plays a big role in the aging process, turning our juicy, plumlike cells into dried-up, wrinkly prunes. Chapter 19 addresses some of the other ways to restore proper hydration levels in your body again, including colon therapy, which helps cleanse your cells of toxins.

The next chapter will look at condiments—those embellishments we tend to ignore—and some of their remarkable healing properties.

CHAPTER 13

HEALING CONDIMENTS:
Delicious and Age Defying

Healthful, high-quality condiments can mean the difference between an average meal and an inspiring one. From starter herbs and spices to delicious finishing oils, these culinary niceties should never be left to chance!

We don't typically think of condiments as anything more than flavor-enhancing substances that we add to foods to make them taste better. But many are healthy and life giving! This chapter reviews some of the little-known health secrets of a few of our favorite condiments.

Apple-Cider Vinegar

Apple-cider vinegar is rich in potassium and helps reestablish a healthy inner ecosystem with friendly bacteria. Thanks to apple-cider vinegar's mineral content (especially potassium), it has the ability to normalize your body's acid/alkaline balance. Its antiseptic qualities cleanse the digestive tract. The acidity aids in the removal of calcium deposits from joints and blood vessels, but has no effect on normal calcium levels in the bones or teeth. Pectin in unfiltered apple-cider vinegar promotes elimination and healthy bowels. The potassium in the vinegar regulates cell growth, hydrates cells, balances sodium, and enables proper performance of the nervous system.

Sipping on a glass of apple-cider vinegar and water during a meal will help increase stomach acid.

Vinegar is also linked to satiety—the feeling of being full. Researchers at the Department of Food Technology, Engineering and Nutrition at Sweden's Lund University recently reported on a study in which 12 healthy subjects ate four "meals" of white wheat bread. One of the meals consisted of bread alone (a control meal), while the others were supplemented with different amounts of vinegar: 18, 23, and 28 grams. Each meal was separated by a week, and each was eaten in the morning after an overnight fast. For two hours, at specific intervals after each meal, subjects rated their feelings of satiety, and researchers took several blood samples from each subject.

The results: Compared with the control meal, the highest level of vinegar intake (between two and three tablespoons) was associated with significantly lower blood sugar and insulin responses and an increased satiety score.[1]

While you may have seen apple-cider vinegar in the grocery store, it may not be the raw, fermented kind that has so many medicinal benefits. Several different companies manufacture apple-cider vinegar. Some bottles are labeled "filtered," but the recommended kind is labeled "unfiltered." Select unpasteurized apple-cider vinegar, which contains the "mother" of the vinegar (a natural sediment with pectin, trace minerals, beneficial bacteria, and enzymes) that you can see floating at the bottom of the bottle.

Adding one tablespoon of apple-cider vinegar to water (you can add stevia to soften the sharp taste) can help alleviate arthritis, aid digestion, combat a sweet tooth, and balance your body at the first sign of cleansing (when it is overly acidic). In fact, sipping apple-cider vinegar in water can be used as an antidote if you've overindulged in sugar or salt. If you feel as if you're coming down with the flu or have signs that a fever blister is about to break out anywhere on your body, immediately sit down to rest and sip on a glass of water with apple-cider vinegar.

One note of caution: Brush your teeth after drinking water with vinegar, as the acid can slowly eat away at the enamel on your teeth if you don't. Another option is to use a straw to protect your teeth.

Apple-cider vinegar is good for your liver and can help with insulin sensitivity (too much blood sugar). You can use it drizzled on your vegetables and as a dressing. It is just one more way to add the sour taste, and it supplies more of those important beneficial microbiota that the body needs and loves.

Sea Salt

High-quality, mineral-rich sea salt is essential for life and has medicinal value. It is grounding, contractive, and stimulates digestion.

The conventional wisdom calling for avoidance of salt because it raises blood pressure is a grave misunderstanding that surfaced when medical research showed that the "salt" Americans were consuming (in large amounts) did indeed increase blood pressure. But here is where we were duped. We were not actually eating salt. The salt in processed foods and in those dark blue cylindrical containers is so refined that none of the beneficial minerals remain; and it is loaded with additives, including sugar, chemicals, bicarbonate of soda, and preservatives. Perhaps the cute little girl on the package should be replaced with a skull and crossbones.

Salt does not raise blood pressure. If yours is high, ask yourself these questions: "Am I drinking enough water for maximum hydration? Do I drink alcohol and wine, causing further dehydration?" These are usually the true underlying causes of elevated blood pressure.

Because salt has an alkalizing effect, we naturally have an innate desire to sprinkle it on acid-forming foods such as animal protein. In fact, salt is the most alkalizing of all foods and can help correct an over-acid condition in the body.

If I could prepare an evening meal for you, I'd serve an appetizing entrée using a grain-like seed (such as quinoa); a dark green, leafy vegetable (such as kale); and a tasty (naturally salty) ocean-veggie dish (such as arame). Of course, a serving of cultured veggies and a champagne glass of one of Body Ecology's probiotic liquids (such as InnergyBiotic) would accompany your meal. Everything would taste wonderful, I promise. Spices and herbs and a high-quality sea salt (Celtic) would be added during cooking to give the dishes more delicious flavor and medicinal value. There would be a nice "finishing salt" (such as Selina Naturally's Hawaiian Makai Pure Sea Salt) on the table to use as you wish. Your body naturally knows how much salt it needs, and when the salt you sprinkle on your food is of excellent quality, you will flourish upon it.

When using sea salt, listen to your intuition and add just enough of this true salt to make your food taste delicious. This means that the flavors will be enhanced, but your food won't taste "salty."

Naturally occurring sodium is an important mineral for the adrenals—remember those two little organs that are responsible for much of your energy? They naturally crave the minerals that sea salt provides. While this alone won't resolve your mineral deficiency, your craving for salt is a "sign" that you need to add many more minerals to your diet and focus on nourishing your adrenals in other ways as well.

But don't forget the Principle of Balance. If you eat too much salt, you may find that you start to crave expansive sweets, as salt is contracting and your body will always seek balance. Do you remember going to the movies when you were a kid and eating a greasy bag of *salty* popcorn, then rushing back to the concession stand for a *sweet* soda to wash it down? If so, then you are already familiar with the body's built-in urge for balance.

So how do you know how much salt is the right amount for you?

That question is impossible for me to answer because according to the Principle of Uniqueness, your need for salt will be unique for you and will fluctuate. We all require differing amounts of sea salt, so there is no "one size fits all" approach. In the summer you will find you desire less salt, and in the winter you'll be using more, especially if you live in a cold climate. Our need for salt becomes more and more intuitive as we create a healthier body.

Men need more salt than women, and children need the least of all. Babies don't require any additional dietary salt during the first two years of life and can obtain their minerals from the foods they're eating. In fact, too much salt can stunt a baby's growth. This can be seen in Japan, where high-salt diets before the Second World War contributed to shorter, stockier adults. After the war, milk (a more expansive food because of the fat) was introduced into the diet of Japanese children, and the next generation grew much taller.

When a woman's body becomes too contracted from a lot of sea salt, she will have extreme cravings for sugary, sweet foods as it attempts to balance itself. This can even affect her temperament and cause mood swings . . . making her feel uptight and cranky.

A woman should be especially mindful of her salt consumption during her monthly cycle. She should cut way back on the amount of sea salt she eats from the moment she begins to ovulate until the beginning of her period (monthly cleansing). This way her body will relax and easily "open up," expanding ever so slightly to release the uterine lining. When a woman eats too much sea salt during her monthly cleansing, she can become too contracted, perhaps bringing to a halt this important opportunity to shed the lining and even eliminate toxins. After the lining is shed and her period is over, she can increase her use of sea salt and contracting foods a bit. Doing so helps the ovary contract and release the tiny egg smoothly at ovulation.

What's in *Your* Shaker?

Buy the best-quality sea salt available—one that retains the high percentage of minerals, trace elements (including iodine), and nutrients that are inadequately represented in our diets today. Minerals, in particular, balance the sodium and chloride in our bodies, and they can't be found in traditional refined salt. A plethora of sea salts are available on the market today, but not all are equal. The ones used in Body Ecology recipes are from *Selina Naturally* (**www.selinanaturally .com**).

Selina DeLangre, who has followed in the footsteps of her father-in-law, Jacques DeLangre, owns Selina Naturally. More than 30 years ago, Jacques founded the Celtic Sea Salt Company and introduced the original brand of Celtic sea salt to Americans. From his own study of the human biological terrain, Jacques realized that we were consuming the wrong type of salt, not only for flavor but also for optimal health. The premium *sel de mer* from Brittany, France, was made famous through his efforts, and he established the standards that all other sea salts with that name attempt to duplicate.

The Truth about Sea Salt and Iodine

There are many misconceptions today concerning salt and iodine. As Selina DeLangre puts it, "It is my intention to sprinkle the truth about salt out of our shakers."

Because of salt's unfortunate link with hypertension, many people have gone to great lengths to reduce their sodium intake. This has resulted in an iodine-deficient diet. One of the most-often-asked questions about Celtic sea salt and Selina Naturally Hawaiian Makai Pure and Portuguese salts is, "Do they have iodine?"

Selina, who has researched this subject for many years, has been kind enough to share her thoughts:

"Iodine is *not* salt, and all salt does *not* have adequate levels of iodine. In other words, you cannot meet your body's needs for iodine with sea salt alone. You must obtain it from other sources as well. Nor can all salts be measured equally.

"There exists in the public eye (and ear), a huge discrepancy and a confusing conspiracy regarding the facts, probably because the FDA, American Heart Association, and the Surgeon General's office are all proclaiming to the public that one must reduce sodium/salt intake. This stigma has had a detrimental effect—people assume this also means reducing or completely eliminating all salt from their daily diets.

"The confusion resulting from the various claims is understandable—one source states: 'Get your iodine from salt,' while the other states: 'Reduce your sodium intake.' Thus, through the elimination of both substances, we've neglected to accept the importance of each of these sacred substances and how they define our well-being.

"According to Dr. David Brownstein, author of the book *Iodine: Why You Need It, Why You Can't Live Without It*, iodine is a very important nutrient, essential for proper thyroid function and brain development. In addition, he maintains that all glandular tissue, including prostate, breasts, ovaries, and all white blood cells, needs sufficient iodine for optimal health.

"Did you know that only 20 percent of all the salts Americans consume contain this important micronutrient? Did you know that most of the popular 'designer salts' usually do not have iodine in them? The type of commercial table salt to which iodine is added is in itself highly toxic!

"Due to the toxicities we are exposed to on a daily basis, such as bromide, fluoride, pesticides, and chlorine derivatives, we require iodine to assist in purging these from our systems. Many 'iodine-fortified table salts' fall short of the nutritional-recommended levels required (and found) in the diet—particularly if you tend to follow a diet without ocean fish or sea vegetables, low-sodium diets, strict vegan diets, or if you just generally consume a diet high in bakery products (such as breads/pastas) that contain bromide.

"In order to help purge your body of toxic buildup, you must increase your body's iodine levels. Be mindful and proactive in helping your body get rid of its toxins. Create more energy so that your body has the strength to detox, drink plenty of water to help move out the toxins, eat antioxidant-rich foods (fermented foods and liquids), take antioxidant supplements like vitamin C, and cleanse your digestive tract with colon therapy. But also consume sea salt, and take **an additional iodine supplement.** It must be unbleached, unrefined, pure sea salt."[i]

[i]Information on iodine provided by Selina DeLangre in conversation with Donna Gates, March 1, 2010.

Selina Naturally Celtic Sea Salt is unprocessed whole salt from one of the most pristine coastal regions of France, harvested by salt farmers using the same method employed by the ancient Celts more than 2,000 years ago. This farming method preserves the purity and balance of ocean minerals. It also contains no anticaking agents, bleaching agents, or other additives.

With the same dedication and passion as Jacques, Selina has developed an exciting selection of salts from natural sources around the world. They can be purchased in health-food stores or from **www .selinanaturally.com.** Look for Celtic, Portuguese (a very light and delicious "finishing" salt), and Hawaiian salt; and Organic Herb Blends made with Celtic sea salt. Today, more than 600 medical professionals use and recommend the Selina Naturally brand.

Herbs and Spices

Herbs and spices are a great way to add flavor and medicinal properties to your meals. Organic varieties are widely available now. Body Ecology has always promoted their use as medicinal healing foods; and now research is showing that the phytochemicals in some spices can actually help with inflammatory diseases such as cancer, diabetes, Crohn's, multiple sclerosis, asthma, arthritis, allergies, Alzheimer's, psoriasis, and AIDS. Spices mentioned in the studies are ginger, basil, rosemary, garlic, red pepper, cloves, anise, fennel, tumeric, and pomegranate.[2]

Other great options are bay leaves, chives, coriander, dill, Italian and Mexican seasonings, mustard powder, marjoram, oregano, black pepper, poppy seeds, sage, tarragon, thyme, nutmeg, and cinnamon.

Garlic—Give It a Place of Honor in Your Pantry

Garlic has been around, well, forever! It is noted in 4,000-year-old Sumerian cuneiform records and is depicted on the walls of ancient Egyptian tombs. It is mentioned in the Bible as a staple of the wandering tribes of Israel. In America, the early colonists became interested in garlic after they noticed how Native Americans used it to treat everything from intestinal worms to scurvy to snakebite.[i]

Chock-full of minerals and nutrients, garlic has powerful antibiotic, antifungal, anticancer, antiparasitic, antioxidant, and antiviral properties. Nearly all cultures attest to its amazing healing potential, and it has been used to treat a wide range of ailments, from athlete's foot to typhoid. New clinical trials are showing that garlic is effective in preventing cancers of the digestive system, including esophagus, stomach, colon, and rectum.[ii]

In fact, some people believe garlic should be classified as a drug. If you know someone who eats garlic regularly and rarely gets sick, it may be because of its special ability to heal wounds both on the inside and outside of the body.

Culinary garlic originated in central Asia, but it was transferred to many other cultures. It does not grow wild today, but was one of our first cultivated plants. As far back as the 1st century A.D., Dioscorides, the Greek physician to Emperor Nero's army, stated that garlic "clears the arteries and opens the mouth of the veins." Two thousand years later, science confirms that garlic is, indeed, a blood thinner or anticoagulant, and protects against heart disease by lowering blood pressure.[iii]

Chewing, chopping, or crushing garlic causes a natural ingredient in the plant called *alliin* to change into the antibiotic substance *allicin*. When garlic cells are ruptured by cutting, they release an enzyme called *allinaise*, which chemically changes the inherent alliin into allicin, and is once again being prescribed by doctors as a treatment for colds and bronchitis. Like chili peppers and other hot foods, garlic works by turning on the body's natural "firefighting faucets" to cool the heat. This prompts the lungs and bronchial tubes to produce more fluids, which in turn thins the mucus and helps flush it out of the body.[iv]

In Ayurvedic medicine, garlic is one of the few foods thought to embody five of the six tastes. The only one it lacks is sour . . . perhaps we should try fermenting it!

---

[i]"Glorious Garlic," from *Optimal Diet* website, **http://homodiet.netfirms.com/ otherssay/letters/garlic.htm**, October 4, 2003, adapted from *Healing Foods from the Bible,* by Bernard Ward (accessed 3/4/10).

[ii]Lisa Fayed, "Garlic and Cancer: Can Garlic Prevent Cancer?" **http://cancer .about.com/od/prevention/a/preventgarlic.htm**, updated May 25, 2006 (accessed 3/4/10).

[iii]Christopher Hobbs, "Garlic: The Pungent Panacea," 1998, from **http://www .christopherhobbs.com/website/library/articles/article_files/garlic_01 .html** (accessed 3/4/10).

[iv]Vitamins & Health Supplements Guide website, **http://www.vitamins-supplements.org/herbal-supplements/garlic.php** (accessed 3/4/10).

Here are some delicious brand-name seasonings with herbs:

- Sea Seasonings Dulse, Dulse with Garlic, Nori with Ginger, and Kelp with Cayenne

- Herbamare (blend of herbs and sea salt)

- Trocomare (blend of herbs, sea salt, and cayenne pepper)

Experiment with your favorite herbs and spices as you try various recipes. You can have a new taste experience just about every day as you vary what you cook and how you flavor it.

Fiber

As you've learned from reading thus far, healthy digestion is essential to feeling your best—and fiber goes a long way toward facilitating this process. Fiber feeds healthy microbes and provides bulk so that as food moves through your digestive tract, cleansing is greatly enhanced. Fiber is also very important because it helps the colon to hold water long enough for maximum hydration.

There are two kinds of fiber—*soluble* and *insoluble.* Most vegetables are about two-thirds soluble, while fruits are about one-third, so they contain a nice balance of both.

Soluble fiber is fiber that dissolves in water. It can have an almost gelatinous quality, and that's why it makes you feel full and satiated after consuming it. Soluble fiber slows down the absorption of nutrients in the small intestine and also functions as a food for short-chain fatty acids, such as *butyrate,* which your cells use as a fuel for keeping the colonocytes (colonic epithelial cells) functioning optimally. These colon cells need to be healthy and strong because they're being exposed to large amounts of free radicals, as well as microbial by-products and toxins found in semisoft and solid bowel movements that are in close and constant contact with the colonic lining.

Insoluble fiber has great value for digestion. It actually pushes against the muscular receptors of the colon and allows for normal peristalsis. Without enough insoluble fiber, your bowel movement becomes small and hard. The colon has to contract harder to move it. Over time this will predispose people to *diverticulosis*—small pouches in the lining of the colon or large intestine that bulge outward through weak spots. When these pouches become inflamed, it can result in a condition called *diverticulitis,* which can lead to bleeding, infections, and small perforations or blockages in the colon.

The other great value of insoluble fiber is that it binds up everything—from fungal toxins to bacteria to heavy metals—that we ingest all the time. The extra bulk in insoluble fiber helps transport these pathogens out in large and healthy bowel movements.

If you're on a plant-based, high-fiber diet and you're well hydrated, you should enjoy healthy eliminations all the time. The Body Ecology program is 80 percent plant based, so it offers many good sources of fiber.

Chia Seeds

Long used by Native Americans in the Southwest for their medicinal and nutritional benefits, chia seeds are rich in omega-3s and omega-6s, calcium, and antioxidants. The soluble fiber in chia seeds is an excellent source of energy and provides a steady release of glucose into the bloodstream. In fact, just one ounce of chia seeds contains 43 percent of your daily fiber! This is great for stamina and strength.

Psyllium, Flax, and Chicory Inulin (FOS)

You may be familiar with psyllium or bentonite as a bulking agent for colon cleansing. These substances virtually pull impacted waste material off the colon walls. When using psyllium, it's crucial to drink a lot of water. Actually, at Body Ecology we try to steer people away from psyllium because it can cause constipation unless you wash it through with at least eight glasses of water per day. We prefer gentler products such as ground flax fiber and EcoBloom (both found in Vitality SuperGreen), along with chia seeds. Plant foods provide the kind of fiber that your body loves best.

Research on flax fiber shows that it protects your colon from cancer and is antiviral, antibacterial, and antifungal. The Body Ecology grain-like seeds, soaked and cooked for a long time, porridge-style, also provide excellent stimulation to the intestines, helping to create a really healthy stool.

Chicory inulin (FOS) is another great form of fiber that also acts as a "prebiotic" food for the healthy bacteria in your system. Chicory inulin helps your body remain hydrated. You may see it listed as an ingredient in several products in health-food stores, and Body Ecology has a product that contains it called EcoBloom. FOS also supports your immune system and helps maintain a healthy cholesterol level. Inulin is a good companion with dairy foods and other products that are high in calcium because it assists calcium absorption.

Fiber has been removed from fruit and vegetable juices, flour products, and most processed foods on the market today. Keep this in mind as you plan how you will eat. Choosing foods that are in their natural form, with fiber intact, goes a long way toward achieving and maintaining optimal health.

Finishing Oils

When you eat the Body Ecology way, oils pressed from olives, nuts, and seeds are used as flavorful toppings to add taste, subtlety, and variety to many dishes.

— **Olive oil:** Extra-virgin olive oil can be drizzled onto everything on your plate. Meat, fish, eggs, vegetables, and grain-like seeds all complement this almost sacred oil. Use it generously and watch your skin grow moist with each passing day. It's an anti-aging miracle.

— **Flaxseed oil:** Use flaxseed oil in salad dressings and mixed into smoothies or as a dip for veggies and bread. Always buy flaxseed oil from a refrigerator case at your health-food store.

— **Pumpkin-seed oil:** This delicious oil adds a nutty flavor when drizzled over salads and veggies or stirred into milk kefir.

— **Macadamia-nut oil:** This is another flavorful alternative to olive oil and has been linked to appetite suppression. Use it as you would any other condiment.

— **Walnut oil:** Produced in California, famous for growing the world's best walnuts, this flavorful oil is perfect for salads, pasta, grilled meats, baking, or just on its own with bread. La Tourangelle produces walnut oil following the traditional method of their French parent company in order to achieve a delicate roasted-walnut taste. Walnut oil is rich in select fatty acids that are essential to human health. The French not only use their precious *huile de noix* as a superb alternative to extra-virgin olive oil for an impressive vinaigrette, but they also love walnut oil over fresh vegetables or drizzled over hard cheeses from the Alps, like comté or emmental. For a unique flavor, try cooking eggs, sautéed chicken, or liver with this exceptional oil. Its rich toasted flavor and incredible nutty aroma will win you over to the point that you will never let your cabinet be without walnut oil again. This oil captures the natural essence and flavor of the nut.

Note: Ideally, avoid cooking with these seed and nut oils, as they are unstable at high heats, become toxic, and their nutritional value is destroyed. As with all oils, store in a cool, dry place (away from the stove!). Flaxseed oil should always be refrigerated (or frozen) to extend its shelf life.

What about Salad Dressing?

A very simple blend of apple-cider vinegar and extra-virgin olive oil, salt, and pepper is an excellent everyday dressing.

For a change of pace, check out Cindy's Kitchen (**www.cindys kitchen.com**), which makes an organic dressing of creamy miso, high-oleic sunflower oil, and extra-virgin olive oil. This is the only Body Ecology–approved dressing on the market so far. A dressing with *refined* sunflower oil would not have obtained our approval, but this one contains *high-oleic* sunflower oil, created by crossbreeding the sunflower plant so that the oil in the seed has a higher percentage of monounsaturated (oleic) fatty acids—similar to olive oil. High-oleic sunflower oil is also less susceptible to destruction by oxygen than regular sunflower oil, another beneficial attribute.

A Healthy Twist on Two Favorites

— **Mustard:** Mustard made with apple-cider vinegar makes a sweet and tangy condiment that is a great topping to turkey burgers. Add it as an ingredient in your salad dressing. A quick recipe appears on the next page.

Mustard Sauce

1 Tbsp. Dijon-style mustard
1 tsp. dry mustard
8–10 drops stevia liquid concentrate
2 Tbsp. apple-cider vinegar
½ cup olive oil (or 1/4 cup olive and 1/4 cup flaxseed oil)
½ cup chopped fresh dill, or 1 tsp. dried

Whisk the Dijon, dry mustard, stevia, and vinegar together in a medium-size bowl. Slowly add the oil, continuing to whisk the mixture until it is thick and well blended. Stir in the dill. Cover and refrigerate at least 1 hour.

— **Mayonnaise, with grapeseed oil:** If you're not into making your own, the only recommended store-bought mayonnaise is from Follow Your Heart. Read the label carefully and choose the one that contains grape-seed oil. (The company has other varieties of mayonnaise.) This egg-free mayo is great for vegans and uses minimally refined grape-seed oil (known for its cholesterol-lowering and anti-oxidant effects). Mayonnaise, diluted with a little water, makes an excellent salad dressing when combined with roasted pumpkin-seed oil, mustard, dulse flakes, sea salt, and a pinch of cayenne.

So, we are ending our discussion of foods appropriately with a culinary "flourish"! I hope you will enjoy experimenting with the wide variety of delicious condiments available on the Body Ecology anti-aging program.

CHAPTER 14

WHERE TO BEGIN:
A Day in the Life of the Body Ecology Program

A very important aspect of digestion is eating the right foods at the right times.

In this chapter you'll find some simple guidelines for how to get started with Body Ecology's way of eating, and the kinds of foods that work best at different points in the day.

Morning

When we wake up in the morning, our bodies are dehydrated, contracted, and naturally acidic. We also need energy to start our day. With the Principle of Balance to guide us, it will be best to drink liquids that hydrate us while giving us energy, that relax us a little, and that also help us become more alkaline. Our bodies are still waking up and need time to get into full gear, so nutritionally dense, easy-to-digest, liquidy foods and drinks are a must.

What would the perfect beginning to the day look like?

First, drink several glasses of water. Nothing hydrates like water, and water with minerals added to help alkalize is best.

Then, drink a "probiotic juice" that acts as an adrenal tonic and also provides the "sweet taste" you need when you are too contracted.

Choose a sour juice such as cranberry, pomegranate, açaí, noni, mangosteen, or black currant; and put this into a probiotic liquid, like young coconut kefir or InnergyBiotic. Add stevia to sweeten.

A cup of an energizing green tea sweetened with stevia, accompanied by a grapefruit sprinkled with sugar-free Lakanto, is comforting on a cold winter's day. Kiwi or a handful of berries provides more energy and antioxidants as you begin your day.

Stir Body Ecology's Vitality SuperGreen or Super Spirulina Plus into some young coconut kefir, and add some chia seeds. Let this thicken for several minutes and you have a great drink that will nurture your intestines.

I always find time to mix a half teaspoon or more of Body Ecology's Super Spirulina Plus (fermented protein powder) into InnergyBiotic. In minutes my energy increases even more.

You can whip up a delicious yet nutritious anti-aging "Green Morning Smoothie" with water, two stalks of celery, two leaves of romaine lettuce, a small zucchini, a small cucumber, some soaked chia seeds, a handful of mint, a large squirt of Barlean's 3-6-9 Swirl Essential Oil, and a few drops of stevia. It's an amazing, alkalizing, high-fiber drink, too.

If your body likes casein (the main protein in dairy foods), pour some homemade milk kefir over a bowl of your favorite berries. Milk kefir is a European favorite in the hot summer months because it is cooling. This cooling quality is great to combat inflammation (internal heat) all year round and is another reason why it is an anti-aging food. Or take the berries and your freshly made milk kefir and add stevia to create a delicious berry smoothie. Milk kefir, a splash of roasted pumpkin-seed oil, some vanilla flavoring, and Lakanto and/or stevia is another tasty smoothie combination.

This light yet extremely nourishing start to your day is a perfect example of practicing calorie restriction with optimal nutrition. These are all good options that hydrate, give you energy, are filling, and are properly combined. An acidic meal is inappropriate, so bacon, eggs, toast, oatmeal, and cereal with milk (a food-combining nightmare) are not part of the Body Ecology Way of Life.

While all the suggestions above are easy to digest, you may want to take digestive enzymes if you feel you need them. For example, even though fermenting helps with digestion of the casein in milk kefir, it may still be difficult for those with weak digestion. If you have this problem, try taking a digestive enzyme with HCl and pepsin to promote digestion of casein in your stomach, and a second enzyme with pancreatin that breaks it down when it reaches your small intestine.

Midday Meals

The best time of the day to eat heavier proteins (such as animal proteins and nut and seed pâtés) is between 11 A.M. and 2 P.M. Your liver is ready to accept proteins at this time, and you are more active and need the extra concentrated energy. Many of us would benefit from eating two smaller protein meals. For example, around 11 A.M., eggs, cultured vegetables, and a small leafy-green salad make for an energizing brunch. Eggs are great for your thyroid and your brain (especially important for a woman when pregnant) and help create energy. At 1 P.M., have a tasty protein-and-veggie lunch served with a small champagne glass of CocoBiotic.

Afternoon Snack

If you need or want to gain weight, have an energizing, alkaline snack such as Vitality SuperGreen or Super Spirulina Plus mixed into young coconut kefir around 3 or 4 P.M. This will give you a midafternoon boost of energy to get you through that period when you feel a bit sleepy or unfocused. Satisfying those afternoon cravings with something healthy will give you more motivation to prepare an evening meal that is balanced and unrushed.

Final Meal of the Day

Your last meal of the day should be vegetarian. Your digestive tract starts to slow down around sunset, so difficult-to-digest, complex meals are not wise. Eat early, and have a light vegetarian meal. You've had a busy day, and it won't be long before you will want to prepare for a great, rejuvenating night of deep sleep. You'll sleep better and awaken refreshed if your last meal is 80 percent vegetables, with a gluten-free grain-like seed such as quinoa, millet, buckwheat, or amaranth.

Now you have everything you need to start your "youthening" food program right away. But growing younger is not just about food—which is why Part III of this book offers some innovative anti-aging strategies. A few may already be a part of your health routine, but others will be exciting new discoveries for you as you continue on your journey toward a longer, healthier life.

PART III

ANTI-AGING THERAPIES FOR EVERYONE

CHAPTER 15

VITAMIN D:
Simple Nourishment from the Sun

It's one of the simplest things—sunlight—but it gives us so much nourishment. Too often we take this everyday element for granted, ignoring its power to heal and replenish our bodies and minds!

Sunshine is as vital to our health as food, oxygen, and water. Certain ultraviolet rays (UVBs) help us make vitamin D, a potent anti-aging hormone and powerful nutrient that offers us countless health benefits. Anthropologists now believe that the pigmentation in our skin actually became lighter as an evolutionary mechanism to acquire more vitamin D when our ancestors migrated away from the equator.

The health benefits of vitamin D fill volumes of scientific journals, and its current widespread deficiency has been identified as a serious epidemic in the U.S., showing up in 80 percent of people of all ages—even newborns. This deficiency will cause us to age quickly . . . very ironic when most of us have been told to avoid the sun because of those ugly brown sunspots and wrinkles. This is why it is so important today to use sunlight wisely, which means obtaining moderate amounts *directly on the skin* and also taking vitamin D supplements.

Your body begins making vitamin D when the UVB rays of the sun react with the 7-dehydrocholesterol in your skin. However, vitamin D does not become a useful hormone until it travels via your bloodstream into the liver to become 25-vitamin D. It then travels on to enter your kidneys and become the active form of vitamin D called 1,25-dihydroxyvitamin D_3, also known as calcitriol or 1,25-DHCC.

Presence of vitamin D signals your intestines to absorb calcium from your diet to build strong bones and teeth. (Please note that the health of your liver and kidneys is important for making vitamin D.)

Researchers at first believed that the kidneys made all the active vitamin D needed by the body, but by the mid-1990s studies began to show that cells in other organs create active vitamin D as well. In other words, the cells in your brain, lungs, colon, and breasts or prostate make it, too. Your brain cells, for example, take up 25-OH vitamin D, convert it into 1,25 vitamin D (the active form), and then consume it.

Vitamin D's importance to our overall health is indisputable. It has now become one of the most intensely studied hormones. A deficiency is serious and well worth your immediate attention.

Why Are We Afraid of the Sun?

As with many of today's health fads, sunlight phobia is a fairly recent phenomenon. We evolved in the sun, and our ancestors embraced and honored it for its life-giving qualities—some even worshipped the sun as God.

It is probably no coincidence that as people grow older, they tend to gravitate to warmer, sunnier climates such as Florida, California, and Arizona. Perhaps intuitively we know that to stay young and healthy, we need even more of the anti-aging hormone it produces in us. Yet the American Academy of Dermatology, well funded by the sunscreen industry, has created so much fear of the sun that many of us never go outside, or only go out wearing chemical-laden, potentially cancer-causing sunscreens.[1]

The Big D—It's Not Just for Bone Health

We have known for a long time that vitamin D plays an important role in bone health, but it does so much more. In fact, it can be called a natural "gene therapy" because it positively influences the functions of at least 2,000 genes. Every tissue and cell recognizes, and has a vitamin D receptor (VDR) for, active vitamin D, even the white blood cells in the immune system. When 1,25-DHCC links to its VDR and then moves into the nucleus of the cell, then the correct programming of these vitamin D—related genes begins. Like a piano player who touches certain keys, it is the selective activation of these genes that determines the overall status of the immune system and its control of inflammation.

This helps explain why vitamin D is a potent weapon against osteoporosis, diabetes, rheumatoid arthritis, multiple sclerosis (MS), high blood pressure, inflammation, Sjögren's syndrome, and thyroid infection. There is also an unmistakable connection between vitamin D deficiency and breast, prostate, and colorectal cancers. You'll notice that all these diseases typically occur later in life.

Immunity

By strengthening our natural immunity and protecting us from viruses, bacteria, and fungal infections that cause inflammation, vitamin D prevents and helps heal inflammatory skin autoimmune conditions, like psoriasis and dermatitis. This is true for types of intestinal inflammation such as IBS, Crohn's disease, and ulcerative colitis as well. Vitamin D also inhibits dangerous autoimmune reactions, where the body turns on itself, as in the case of Hashimoto's disease, a disease of the thyroid gland.[i]

Muscle Mass

Essential for maintaining muscle mass throughout life, vitamin D helps preserve the Type II muscle fibers that are prone to atrophy in older people. In addition, recent research reveals an association between higher vitamin D levels and improved physical functioning as we age.[ii]

Heart Disease

Researchers from the University of Warwick, England, evaluated 28 studies involving almost 100,000 men and women across different ethnic groups. The data revealed a strong association between high levels of vitamin D and significantly lower risk of both cardiac and metabolic disorders. Compared to those with low levels, men and women who had high levels of vitamin D had a reduced risk of developing cardiovascular disease by about 33 percent, elevated blood sugar by 55 percent, and metabolic syndrome by more than 50 percent.[iii] Vitamin D also regulates insulin secretion by the pancreas and may increase insulin sensitivity better than some diabetic drugs such as Metformin.[iv]

Weight Loss

Vitamin D and sunlight should be included in any successful weight-loss program. Believe it or not, even your fat cells have receptor sites for vitamin D. Give them adequate amounts and they become more active and burn up calories more efficiently. Also, your fat cells secrete a hormone called leptin that tells the brain when you are full. A deficiency of vitamin D prevents this hormone from working well so that you are less able to control your appetite.

---

[i]M. D. Griffin, N. Xing, and R. Kumar, "Vitamin D and its analogs as regulators of immune activation and antigen presentation," *Annual Review of Nutrition*, 23 (2003): 117–145. (First published online as a Review in Advance on March 19, 2003.)

[ii]"Vitamin D Status Associated with Physical Function in Older Men and Women," *Life Extension*, April 30, 2010, **http://www.lef.org/newsletter/2010/0430_Vitamin-D-Associated-with-Physical-Function-in-Older-Men-Women .htm?source=eNewsLetter2010Wk18-2&key=Archive** (accessed 10/6/10).

[iii]J Parker, O. Hashmi, D. Dutton, A. Mavrodaris, S. Stranges, N. B. Kandala, A. Clarke, and O. H. Franco, "Levels of vitamin D and cardiometabolic disorders: Systematic review and meta-analysis," *Maturitas,* 65(3) (March 2010): 225–236, as found in article by Allen S. Josephs, M.D., "Vitamin D Continues to Dominate," **Vitacost.com** website, February 24, 2010, **http://www.vitacost.com/ Vitamin-D-Continues-to-Dominate-printable?csrc=EM-FYH20100225:print** (accessed 10/6/10).

[iv]K. C. Chiu, A. Chu, V. Liang W. Go, and M. F. Saad, "Hypovitaminosis D is associated with insulin resistance and ß cell dysfunction," *American Journal of Clinical Nutrition,* 79 (May 2004): 820–825.

Only the negative effect of UV rays is presented to the public. Yes, *chronic* or *excessive* exposure does, indeed, increase the risk of nonmelanoma (basal- or squamous-cell) cancers, but these types of skin cancer rarely spread, are rarely lethal, and can be easily removed by surgery.

There is very little evidence that the potentially deadly form of skin cancer, melanoma, is caused by *sensible* amounts of sun exposure. In fact, new research indicates that sensible amounts *decrease* the risk of cancers, including melanoma, by controlling cell growth and inducing cells that are malignant to become normal or to die of apoptosis (programmed death). While skin-cancer cases total about one million per year in the U.S., they are lethal in only about 2,000 cases, which is only .5 percent of all cancer deaths.[2]

Vitamin D regulates up to 200 genes that control cell growth and cellular differentiation, so it is not surprising that it prevents up to 16 other types of deadly cancer that *do* spread and *do* kill. So the benefits of the sun may far outweigh the small risk of skin cancer.

To harness the power of the sun safely, it's important to understand the difference between UVA and UVB rays. UVA rays penetrate deeply, and when you are out in the sun too long, they have a negative effect on the elasticity of the skin. They cause wrinkles and brown or white pigmentation, sometimes called sunspots. UVA rays are the major cause of the potentially lethal melanomas. UVB rays, on the other hand, redden and can potentially burn the skin, but are the only rays that make vitamin D. Over time, without proper protection from sunburn, UVB rays can cause skin cancer. Once again, it's a matter of prudent sun exposure.

Sun Sensitivity . . . Could Our Poor Diets Be a Clue?

What explains our hypersensitivity to the sun these days? After all, skin cancers were at one time fairly uncommon.

Remember, the first step in making vitamin D begins when the sun reacts with a type of cholesterol in your skin. Dietary fats and oils affect the quality of cholesterol in your body.

Our supersensitivity to the sun seems to coincide with the dietary changes that occurred at the beginning of the 20th century when we began eating fats and oils that were heated, refined, bleached, and deodorized. Instead of having small amounts of healthy, vitamin D–rich raw butter and ghee, we've been consuming margarine and trans fats for generations. The liver, which plays a key role in producing vitamin D, is also damaged by toxic fats and oils.

Even as you begin eating the recommended healthy fats and oils, poor *absorption* of dietary fats becomes another concern. Your liver and gallbladder may be in need of special care and attention, and your digestion of fats (which occurs in your small intestine) may be inadequate and will contribute to low levels of vitamin D.

The good news is that a probiotic diet, with lots of fermented foods, will improve the health of your liver and gallbladder and greatly assist in your digestion of fats. As the beneficial microbiota work to keep your intestines optimally functioning, your liver benefits as well.

How Much Vitamin D Is the Right Amount?

This is an area of much controversy, and there is a lot of negative information floating around on the Internet. With so much confusion, it is smart to turn to the experts out there who are doing the cutting-edge research, people like Dr. Michael Holick and Dr. John Cannell.

Dr. Holick's informative book, *The Vitamin D Solution: A 3-Step Strategy to Cure Our Most Common Health Problem* (Penguin/Hudson Street Press, 2010), is an excellent place to turn for credible information and a list of charts that tell you how long to expose yourself to the sun depending on where you live and the color of your skin. Dr. Holick is the scientist who discovered the active form of vitamin D and has worked closely with other experts in his field uncovering the truth about this essential anti-aging hormone. See his website: **www .vitamindhealth.org.**

Also, it would be wise and commendable to join (and financially support) Dr. Cannell's nonprofit organization, called the Vitamin D Council (**www.vitamindcouncil.org**). This way you can stay updated on the fascinating and extensive research being done around the world. If you spend time on his website, you will be thoroughly convinced that vitamin D is for you. Dr. Cannell sends out a free educational newsletter.

Both Cannell and Holick are comfortable recommending at least 5,000 IUs per day of a vitamin D supplement (for an adult). After testing, you may want to increase the amount to 10,000 IUs per day. However, evidence is mounting that even higher levels may be needed by many of us. The larger amounts are important if you have not been out in the sun or have signs of osteopenia, osteoporosis, or cancer.

If you are overweight, you will need to take more (perhaps twice as much) because vitamin D gets locked into fat cells and cannot be released. Anyone with intestinal disorders, like Crohn's disease, inflammation problems, or diarrhea, requires larger amounts, and supplements may not be useful at all. (See the "Tanning Beds?" section later in this chapter.)

Can you take too much vitamin D in supplement form? This is a hotly debated subject among researchers today, and many currently believe that you can. (You can never overdose on vitamin D made from sunlight or food.) Symptoms of vitamin D toxicity (from taking too much from a supplement) include nausea, loss of appetite, vomiting, and elevated blood pressure. If you experience these problems and excessive supplementation continues, you could suffer kidney failure.

Currently, however, your doctor will want you to reach blood levels of 54–90 nanograms per milliliter (ng/ml) of blood. These numbers are ones to watch, though, as newer research suggests that levels of 80–90 ng/ml are even better. (Lifeguards often have levels as high as 100–200 ng/ml.) If you want to rejuvenate and experience greater vitality, then levels in the low 30s (which some doctors consider to be sufficient) will be grossly inadequate.

As extensive, worldwide research continues to unfold, it's still not clear what the precise "ceiling" vitamin D levels might be. However, levels higher than were originally thought safe are now proving to be quite harmless and even beneficial (even up to 200 ng/ml) as long as simple blood tests show that your parathyroid hormone levels and your calcium-to-phosphorus ratio remain normal.

You can obtain your own levels of vitamin D by visiting your doctor or by ordering an inexpensive blood-test kit from the Vitamin D Council website, or from **www.zrtlab.com.** (You should retest three or four times per year.) Blood levels do change. If your levels are high at the end of the summer, they may be quite low in the winter, so retest. Given that new information on the benefits of vitamin D, as well as the recommended blood level and supplement dosage, is being compiled monthly, choose a doctor who is up-to-date on the latest research. Also, joining Dr. Cannell's nonprofit will keep you current. As new guidelines become available, you'll be one of the first to know.

A Supplement Isn't Enough . . . Embrace the Sun

A supplement alone isn't sufficient if you are truly serious about rejuvenation. Vitamin D from sunlight remains in the body at least twice as long as that derived from diet. What's more, there are unique substances in sunlight, called "photoproducts," that you cannot obtain from food or a supplement. Scientists, including Dr. Holick's group, are now looking carefully at these photoproducts, feeling certain that if they are there, it must be for a biological reason.

You'll definitely feel happier from sunlight. Research shows that when you go into the sun, keratinocytes in your skin cells actually create endorphins, which improve feelings of well-being.

Exposure to the sun helps regulate our circadian rhythms. We sleep better and are far less likely to suffer from depression and seasonal affective disorder (SAD). (Supplements do not improve circadian rhythm.)

What Is "Prudent" Sun Exposure?

You should never go into the sun and get burned. Start sunbathing for short periods at first, and slowly and carefully build up a base tan. Prior to the Industrial Revolution, working outdoors probably helped build a resistance to sunburn. It appears that those who have developed higher vitamin D levels (like roofers and lifeguards) do not burn as easily. Therefore, correcting your vitamin D deficiency with supplements before spending time in the sun might be wise, especially if you are fair-skinned and tend to burn easily.

Midday is the best time to sunbathe because the rays reach us directly. In the morning or afternoon, they are coming in at angle and are not as effective.

Most people can go into the sun starting with 10 minutes at first and then building up to as much as 60 minutes at midday (depending on how intense the sun is in your area). If you must remain outside longer, you should then apply a chemical-free, broad-spectrum sunscreen that shields you from UVA and UVB rays. Badger sunscreen, which is zinc oxide and herbs (no chemicals), was rated the safest sunscreen of more than 600 tested by the Environmental Work Group (**www.ewg.org**). See **www.badgerbalm.com** for more information.

You'll want to protect your face and hands by wearing sunscreen and/or a hat. The less clothing you wear, the more vitamin D your body will make. If you are fortunate enough to live in a sunny region, only 20 minutes in the sun a day will give you what you need. If you are an African American with darker skin, Dr. Holick suggests that you may need as much as three to ten times that amount of exposure.

Tanning Beds?

Tanning beds have been shown to dramatically increase vitamin D levels in the blood. If used properly, they can safely produce vitamin D in the winter months when it is impossible to get enough sun to prevent disease. However, they must be used in moderation and responsibly. Dr. Holick tells his readers to find a facility that has been certified by the International Smart Tan Network. He recommends that you make sure they use low- or medium-pressure fluorescent lamps. He also warns that you must be just as cautious as you would with regular sunlight and protect your face and lips with sunscreen and your eyes with goggles.

If you have an intestinal-absorption problem (due to surgery, Crohn's disease, celiac disease, or diarrhea from infections), you may not respond well to vitamin D supplementation. Tanning beds could be a good alternative for you.

Simple Dietary Secrets That Will Unleash the Power of Vitamin D

Certain nutrients are "cofactors" that are essential for the assimilation of vitamin D. The most important cofactor is magnesium, but your diet and supplements should also include sources of vitamin K_2, zinc, boron, and a small amount of vitamin A. For example, all the enzymes that metabolize vitamin D require magnesium. Basically, vitamin D won't work in the body without it. If you try to elevate your vitamin D levels and are deficient in magnesium, you will only intensify your magnesium deficiency. If, after you take vitamin D, tests show that your levels are not rising, look elsewhere for the problem.

Simply taking your vitamin D supplements with your largest meal of the day may quickly improve your blood levels of D. Researchers at the Cleveland Clinic examined 17 patients who were not getting better under treatment. By taking vitamin D *with* their biggest meal, they boosted the level of vitamin D in their blood by an average of 56 percent.[3]

Sun-dried mushrooms such as dried shiitake (often exposed to extra sunlight during the growing process to create even more vitamin D) are your richest dietary source of this wonder nutrient. Fresh mushrooms don't supply nearly as much, but are still quite good.

Wild or wild-caught salmon and albacore tuna are excellent sources of vitamin D. Farmed salmon never has the vitamin D content of wild or wild-caught salmon. The term *wild-caught* means the salmon are born in hatcheries and released into the wild. Every year in Washington State, elementary-school classes vie for the privilege of performing this task—really! All hatcheries mark these "fry" (the fish, not the kids!) by clipping their fins so they can't be confused with the truly wild salmon.

Sockeye salmon cannot be farmed, so it's your best choice. Atlantic salmon from your local supermarket is always farmed. Canned salmon contains vitamin D but is overcooked and difficult to digest.

Canned sardines, mackerel, and tuna can also provide you with vitamin D. Depending on the brand, cod-liver oil (**www.green pasture.org**) is right up there with wild salmon as a good source of D.

However, upping your intake of cod-liver oil above two tablespoons a day could cause an overdose of vitamin A. Fermented milk kefir, butter, ghee, and egg yolks provide only small amounts of D, so you can't correct a deficiency relying on these alone. Ocean's Alive Marine Phytoplankton (**www.sunfoods.com**) is a high-quality, vegan source of vitamin D.

Please don't think you can get vitamin D from fish-oil capsules. While a potentially excellent source of omega-3 fatty acids (depending on the brand and quality), fish oil does not contain vitamin D.

Remember that vitamin D tells your intestines to absorb more calcium and is essential to the uptake of this mineral in your diet. So increase your dietary calcium by eating plenty of dark green, leafy vegetables such as kale, collards, escarole, bok choy, and Brussels sprouts. Sea vegetables are another excellent source of calcium. Avoid calcium-depleting substances, especially sugar, and too much fruit, alcohol, and caffeine. Drugs like prednisone and diuretics also deplete calcium.

By increasing your intake of vitamin D and calcium, doing resistance exercises that work against gravity (yoga, Pilates, walking, weight training, climbing stairs, or dancing), and making sure you digest your food well (with enzymes and fermented foods and drinks), you are well on your way to creating superhealthy bones that will be resistant to breaks and deterioration as you age.

CHAPTER 16

BREATHWORK:
The Life-Giving Power Inside of You

*Breathing is basic to life. Why, then,
do so many of us breathe so poorly?*

Most of us use only a fraction of our full breathing capacity. Particularly when we're stressed, we breathe from the chest in short, gaspy intakes. Proper breathing should originate from the diaphragm—full, deep, and rhythmic.

Right now, take a long, slow, deep breath. Did your abdomen expand?

Deep abdominal breathing has many benefits for anti-aging. For example, did you know that breathing directly affects your body's pH balance? Poor breathing also results in chronic fatigue, muscle cramps, cold hands and feet, heartburn, PMS, impaired concentration, and more.[1] Proper breathing can help you metabolize your food better and improve your ability to concentrate and remember.

Some people believe that as infants we breathed perfectly. But over time we developed "muscle armoring," beginning with the diaphragm and continuing to the pelvis, chest, back, legs, and throat.[2] These muscular tensions, along with poor posture and self-consciousness about keeping our stomachs flat, compromise the easy, effortless breathing we enjoyed as babies.

There are a number of breathing techniques you might try to dismantle this muscle armoring, including bioenergetics, the Alexander Technique, and various styles of yoga and yoga meditations. Holistic retailers such as Gaiam offer CDs that guide listeners through simple breathing exercises.

With regular practice, breathing correctly will begin to become second nature. You will feel new levels of stamina, as well as improved digestion and elimination. Many people who have practiced deep breathing regularly report that it generates a profound feeling of contentment and alleviates anxiety and nervous tension.

Hyperbaric Oxygen Therapy

Hyperbaric oxygen therapy (HBOT) is a treatment dating back to the 17th century, although it has only been recognized in conventional medicine since the 1940s. It involves breathing 100 percent oxygen while under increased atmospheric pressure. In this way, the oxygen concentration in the body becomes up to 20 times its normal amount at the cellular level. Basically, the increased pressure deposits a lot of oxygen into the blood plasma in all bodily cells, tissues, and fluids.

The treatment, which is painless, consists of lying down on a bed inside a pressure chamber. Patients can sleep or even read while in the chamber—there is no need to wear a hood or a mask. Some people can experience a popping in their ears due to the increase in pressure, similar to what is experienced when changing altitude in airplanes. Chewing gum or swallowing hard can alleviate this.

My friend Raymond Crallé introduced me to HBOT in 2008. Raymond, who has been a practicing physical therapist in Delray Beach, Florida, for 35 years, believes that when HBOT is delivered on a long-term basis, it can slow down the aging process. He uses it in his practice to treat a variety of brain and sports injuries. Ray himself is a testament to the anti-aging benefits of oxygen therapy. He is the proud father of two amazingly calm yet alert and intelligent little girls. His oldest daughter received oxygen from birth. His youngest began doing so while she was in the womb.

In their book, *The Oxygen Revolution,* authors Paul G. Harch and Virginia McCullough argue that hyperbaric oxygen actually acts at the DNA level to stimulate growth and repair hormones. Although HBOT has long been an effective treatment for burn victims and those suffering from decompression sickness, many healers are beginning to see that it has a much more far-reaching impact in promoting natural healing and can be used to treat a wide range of conditions, including Alzheimer's, fibromylagia, viruses, and immune-system disorders. Others, like Harch and McCullough, believe that HBOT can literally rejuvenate our "tired brains," which have suffered chemical and toxic insults over the course of a lifetime that have contributed to premature aging.[3]

As you know by now, according to the Principle of Balance, everything has two sides. We must always look for the negative one so we can balance or fix it. For example, antibiotics have saved millions of lives. But had we known 60 years ago to look for their downside, we might have prevented hundreds of millions of yeast or fungal infections.

What is the drawback of HBOT? Oxygen, while it does much good, also creates more free radicals. Hyperbaric oxygen therapy can stress the liver as well.

So what can be done to undo the negative side effects of HBOT— yet still reap its many benefits? How would you create balance? There are three recommended actions:

1. Increase Antioxidants

Significantly increase the amount of antioxidants you consume during your weeks of therapy. Your diet should include even more of the enzyme-rich fruits and vegetables recommended by Body Ecology. Fermented foods and liquids are the ultimate antioxidants, so consume large amounts.

Increase your levels of glutathione, a master antioxidant. A green shake made of Vitality SuperGreen combined with un-denatured whey-protein concentrate helps increase glutathione. Up the amount of minerals you take in via food and supplements to keep your body more alkaline.

Anti-Aging on the Cutting Edge

Activated Air

Breathing "biophysically altered" air is a way to counter free radicals or oxidative stress. The Active Air device, manufactured by Eng3, can be used at home. A valuable healing and anti-aging tool, it can help strengthen your immune system and accelerate recovery from illness. It is also a great way to create energy.

The Active Air device creates higher levels of oxygen in the body, but it does so in a different way than HBOT. Unlike HBOT, which delivers concentrated air, this technology delivers an oxygen level that is the same as regular air. Because of the free-radical damage done by pressing oxygen into the system, hyperbaric treatments should be considered a short-term solution, while an activated-air machine actually repairs and protects against free-radical damage.

Go to **www.eng3corp.com** to learn more.

2. Cleanse More Actively

Cleansing your colon at this time with home enemas or with a visit to your professional colon therapist is key.

While undergoing HBOT, the mitochondria in your cells receive significantly more oxygen. This increases energy in your body (the positive). But what happens when your energy goes up? Your cells immediately start to cleanse and push *out* toxins. These toxins put a greater burden on your liver (the negative).

Yes, you may be having a healthy elimination each day . . . but this is a time when your body will need to eliminate even more than usual. Colon therapy is wonderful way to create balance.

3. Take Extra Special Care of Your Liver

A mostly raw diet using the Body Ecology principles is appropriate during HBOT because a raw diet is best for the liver. Take care to eat few or no fats or oils at this time, avoiding cooked saturated fats in particular. Take a liver-cleansing supplement such as Body Ecology's LivAmend, which works by increasing bile flow. Bile is produced in your liver, and toxins are dumped into the bile and then sent to your gallbladder. When you eat, this stored bile is deposited into the colon, where it stimulates peristaltic movement so that the toxins can be eliminated with the bowel movement. Because the daily bowel movement is usually not sufficient to remove toxins fast enough, colon cleansing at this time is highly recommended. If you're having a daily HBOT session, then a daily enema or at least four colon-therapy sessions per week is best.

CHAPTER 17

SLEEP:
Your Anti-Aging Ally

*Learning how to maximize rejuvenating sleep
is one of the keys to longevity, happiness, and health.*

Insufficient sleep plagues 50 million to 70 million Americans today, especially women. Yet, sleeping deeply like a newborn baby is crucial for restoring your prenatal jing. It is absolutely fundamental for staying young, healthy, and vibrant. And . . . it's free!

As the years pass, sleep often becomes more elusive. If you are not falling asleep, staying asleep, and waking up on time feeling refreshed, you'll want to change this as soon as possible. The Principle of Step by Step tells you to first and foremost create more energy to heal or to reclaim the vitality you had in your mother's womb. Sleep is one way to do this.

It *must* be important to sleep; there is not an animal on the planet that doesn't do it. A really great night's rest is an investment in your anti-aging bank account. Insufficient sleep is associated with increased risk for diabetes, heart disease, depression, and obesity.

Your brain is very much affected by the *quality* of your sleep. Research clearly confirms what you've probably already observed—your mood, cognition, and memory are negatively affected by sleep deprivation. Notice the vast difference in what you are willing to do for yourself and for others when you've gotten a great night's rest.

In fact, a recent study with university students found that sleep can help you remember something you need to do in the future.

After giving a series of tests to 24 students who slept after processing and storing the idea of a planned task, researchers found that these students were more likely to follow through on their intentions than those who tried to tackle their plan before going to sleep. Researchers believe that this process, called *prospective memory,* occurs during slow-wave sleep (an early pattern in the sleep cycle) and involves communication between the brain's hippocampus (memory formation) and its cortical regions (memory storage).[1]

But it's not only your mood and memory that are impacted by sleep. Your very life depends upon it! The North Carolina DMV's *Driver's Handbook* offers up this little cautionary statistic: "Anyone who has had less than five hours of sleep the night before is four to five times more likely to crash than someone who got eight hours of sleep."[2]

And a team of British and Italian researchers determined that if you regularly sleep less than six hours a night, you are 12 percent more likely to die prematurely. *Chronic insomnia* (the inability to fall asleep or remain asleep for an adequate amount of time) also elevates one's risk of an earlier death. Interestingly, these researchers—after analyzing 16 sleep studies that included more than 1.3 million people—also found that sleeping *too much* (more than nine hours a night) might be an important sign of a serious or potentially fatal illness.[3]

So the solution is to sleep within an optimal range of seven to nine hours every night. But bear in mind, this applies to adults only. Babies and toddlers spend many more hours in sleep a day, around 10 to 14. Children require between 10 and 12, and teenagers need at least 9 hours. By contrast, older adults tend to sleep a little less, to sleep more lightly, and to take more catnaps.[4]

The Mechanics of Sleep

Early in the night, there is a greater amount of slow-wave deep sleep, which is the most restorative sleep. Growth hormone is produced during the initial onset of nightly sleep. Go to bed early and you'll not only become "healthy, wealthy, and wise," but you'll also look and feel younger. Smaller pulses of growth hormone are also released later in your sleep cycle, so if you only sleep for five hours, you won't obtain enough of this rejuvenating hormone.

Rapid eye movement (REM) or "dream" sleep is active sleep—important for the development and health of your brain. REM increases later in the sleep cycle and just before you naturally awaken.

Melatonin, often called the most potent antioxidant in the human body, is critical to restorative sleep. A natural hormone secreted by the pineal gland in your brain, melatonin increases with darkness, causing drowsiness. It then decreases with the morning light, and you begin to wake up. Because the production of this important hormone is suppressed by light, working late into the night, especially on the computer, or watching late-night television might be cutting off years from your life.

Tips for Sleeping Long and Well

Most of us look for shortcuts when it comes to sleep. As with weekend-warrior exercise, we think we can "make up" for weekday deficits by sleeping in on the weekend. But that's not how it works. Here are a few suggestions for restorative sleep:

— **Reset your circadian rhythm.** Get up early and start to move. Try stretching with the ancient yoga posture called the Sun Salutation. A walk in the morning light will help you sleep better that night. In the spring, summer, and fall, sunbathe midday for 20 to 30 minutes.

— **Start to unwind as the evening begins.** Take a Chinese herbal formula called Peaceful Spirit (available from **www.jingherbs .com**). The herbs open your heart, calm your spirit, and relax your nervous system to prepare for the evening ahead. The main ingredient, *reishi,* is often called the "mushroom of immortality" and is also an excellent source of vitamin D. Called their "happy formula" by Jing Herbs, Peaceful Spirit is used as a treatment for sadness and anxiety because another ingredient, *polygala root,* strengthens the connection between your heart (shen) and your adrenals (jing). The Chinese asparagus "puts a wing on your heart."

— **Celebrate sleep.** As bedtime approaches, begin to celebrate the ritual of sleep. Take a hot bath and create a "sleep sanctuary," with soft organic bedding, candles, soothing incense or aromatherapy, gentle music, and the like.

— **Consider herbs.** You may need to take something to help you sleep. Noncaffeinated teas such as chamomile, tulsi, skullcap, and valerian have a mildly sedating effect. In Chinese medicine, the "shen herbs" are calming.

- If you have issues with an overactive mind that won't shut off and let you sleep, Bupleurum & Dragon Bone (also from Jing Herbs) can help. This classic formula has been used for more than 2,000 years with great success. It differs from Peaceful Spirit because it addresses an overactive liver energy that causes inner "chatter." It also moves the energy out of your head and into your heart, where your "spirit resides during sleep," giving you a sense of well-being and of feeling like you are at home in your own skin. Because of the calming and grounding qualities, Bupleurum & Dragon Bone formula is used for insomnia. However, other modern-day applications include anxiety; angina pectoris; and addictive behaviors such as smoking, drinking, drug use, and overeating.

- If you can't sleep because of hot flashes, night sweats, itchiness, and irritability, then Jing Herb's Winter Yin Formula is a modified classic formula for clearing "heat" and for those who have depleted their reserves of energy.

- Melatonin supplements can be purchased at your local health-food store and can help regulate sleep. When taken short-term, melatonin is safe and is especially useful when you travel and change time zones.

Side effects may include morning grogginess, vivid dreams, and a lower body temperature. Melatonin also suppresses your desire for sex. Supplements can be purchased in one- to five-milligram capsules. You will have to experiment to find the best dosage for you. Start with the lowest amount and increase if necessary. Take melatonin 45 minutes before bedtime. Time-released versions may be a better choice if you awaken often during the night.

— **Aim for eight hours of sleep a night.** Some of us will require a little more, while others will function just fine on seven hours if it is quality sleep. Napping works for many, and you may feel the need to take rejuvenating catnaps during the day. (See the "Power Napping" section to follow.) What's most important is that your sleep be restful and restorative, with three to five complete sleep cycles that take you from drowsiness, into light sleep, followed by deep and then deeper sleep, and ending in REM.

— **Eat grain-like seeds in the evening.** Your last meal of the day should have been a calming grain-like seed (quinoa, millet, buckwheat, or amaranth) that helps create more serotonin (which then turns into melatonin).

— **Keep a regular schedule.** Try to go to bed and wake up around the same time. This also helps set your biological clock. A good rule of thumb is to avoid anything that is too "stimulating" before bedtime. That includes alcohol, caffeine, and sugar, which disturb circadian rhythms.

— **Sleep in total darkness.** Light also interferes with production of melatonin, so get rid of the night light in your bathroom or bedroom. Several hours before bed, withdraw from visually stimulating activities like television, the Internet, take-home work, and so on. Vigorous exercise can also be a bit too exciting to the body, leaving you energized rather than calm. Try more soothing kinds of exercise, like yoga or stretching or a leisurely walk, if you need to relieve tension.

Power Napping

Not only is regular and restorative sleep important, research reveals that taking naps can also improve cognitive performance and your ability to absorb new information.

Anti-Aging on the Cutting Edge

The Earthing Pad

Remember free radicals . . . those oxidizing villains that result from chronic stress and environmental toxins? Sixty years ago, we began to wear shoes with synthetic soles and unknowingly lost our connection with the greatest free-radical neutralizer, Mother Earth.

Throughout most of human history, we walked barefoot or slept on the ground. The earth's tranquil energy naturally transfers to any conductive object it is in contact with—whether it is a metal rod, a wire, a tree or plant, an animal, or a barefoot human—and it becomes "grounded." The known effect of grounding is to discharge and prevent the buildup of electrical stress.

Our bodies are mostly water, and minerals are excellent conductors of electricity (electrons). The free electrons on the surface of the planet are easily transferred to the human body as long as there is direct contact. Unfortunately, synthetically soled shoes act as insulators so that even when we are outside, we do not connect with the earth's electric field. When we are in homes and office buildings, we are also insulated and unable to receive the earth's balancing energies.

Having your bare feet touch the ground connects you with an infinite supply of *free* electrons. The Earthing Pad is a unique tool for neutralizing the painful and chronic inflammation that causes autoimmune and degenerative diseases, including aging.

In fact, the patented Earthing technology is the only way, without standing directly on the ground, to connect with Earth's electrons. It allows you to connect to the earth during sleep or while you work. As it neutralizes free radicals in your body, it supports your immune system; reduces stress and anxiety; and is fundamental to sound, restorative sleep. There is no question that maintaining a functionally "young" immune system is an excellent strategy for preserving the quality of life and slowing senescence. As Earthing greatly reduces oxidative stress, it is expected to increase life expectancy and improve health.

To learn much more about this simple but essential healing tool, read *Earthing: The Most Important Health Discovery Ever?* by Clint Ober, Stephen T. Sinatra, M.D., and Martin Zucker.

To purchase an Earthing Pad for your desk or bed, go to **www .longevitywarehouse.com**. The products offered on this website allow you to conveniently ground yourself when indoors. They are "barefoot substitutes."

Everyone in your family should be working and sleeping on an Earthing Pad. An affordable anti-aging tool, it should be under your feet while you are at your computer and on your bed at night.

A study at the University of California–Berkeley recruited 39 healthy adults and assessed their ability to learn and memorize with or without naps. The participants who napped between learning sessions (for 90 minutes) improved their scores by 10 percent, while their non-napping counterparts saw scores dropping by 10 percent.[5] Napping can also be beneficial for those who have insomnia issues or problems with sleep apnea.

Many cultures, especially those in hotter climates, have long known the value of napping . . . think of Spain and their famous afternoon *siestas*. However, in America's corporate culture, it can be a bit more challenging to find time for napping, especially if you work at an office and follow a typical 9-to-5 schedule. You might consider taking a 30-minute nap during your lunch break after you've eaten. Some companies even provide "meditation" rooms for employees who need to "recharge their batteries" for a little while.

The traditional Sunday-afternoon nap, in a favorite armchair or hammock, was once practically an American institution . . . and for many of us who want to stay youthful and young looking, it certainly should become one again!

A Few Things about Napping

- You are an experiment of one, so try taking a few afternoon naps and observe how you feel afterward. If you complain of waking from naps groggy and disoriented, it may be that you have gone into deep sleep (stages 3 and 4), which means you won't wake as easily. But if your nap only takes you through the first two stages of sleep, you will most likely wake up feeling energized and more alert. As the first two stages of sleep take about 10 minutes each, the best napping time is around 20 minutes.[6]

- Don't nap late in the day, as this can interfere with your regular sleep schedule. The prime napping time is between 1 and 3 in the afternoon.

- Try not to nap for more than about 30 minutes. Longer than that may actually have the opposite effect of what you intend, and you may wake feeling tired and listless. You might want to set your watch or phone alarm to make sure you don't "over-nap."

- Try to find a darkened room or use eye pillows or a mask to create daytime darkness. Quiet is essential.

How Do You Know If You Need a Nap?

One method is to sit in a comfortable chair with your feet flat on the floor, back upright but supported by the chair. Then simply breathe into and out of your belly slowly for about five to ten minutes. If you are tired when you do this, you will usually fall asleep. If that happens, lie down or just take a nap in the chair. Even if you don't feel sleepy, you will benefit from the quiet contemplation and deep-breathing exercises. Even taking a mental siesta for ten minutes here and there during the day will improve your outlook and attitude.

Now that we've covered the basics—the anti-aging tools that are part of our birthright—it's time to move on to some truly innovative, cutting-edge approaches to longevity. The next few chapters will highlight the latest and greatest therapies and products in the life-extension field of medicine. We'll start with detoxification therapies—because pure, clean, well-nourished cells are the secret to a long and healthy life.

CHAPTER 18

DETOXIFICATION:
The Secret to Longevity

Pure, clean, well-nourished cells
are the secret to longevity. End of story!

Earlier we learned that one of the principal causes of aging is the buildup and storage of toxins in the body. Unfortunately, many of us begin life on this planet with toxins in our cells. Some we inherited from our parents and grandparents, and even more toxins entered our cells at birth. In fact, up until fairly recently general anesthesia for women in the delivery room was standard practice, and today many women are given other drugs during labor.

As infants, we receive vaccinations, many of which contain mercury. Later, we probably take antibiotics that destroy the beneficial bacteria we need for healthy digestion. And as the years pass, we continue to be assaulted by a "chemical soup" of pollutants—from processed foods to household products. I actually remember one summer when I was nine my brother and I entertained ourselves by taking the mercury from a thermometer, rolling it into a ball, and playing with it—our own version of toxic Play-Doh.

No one knew. . . .

Toxins from the Inside and Out

Many of the toxins that harm us are *exogenous*. They are found in the external environment—our food, water, and air. They are in the pots and pans we cook with, the fillings in our teeth, and the cosmetics we put on our faces. Many of us are experiencing symptoms of heavy-metal toxicity that our overstressed organs of elimination are simply not able to handle.

Other toxins are *endogenous*. They are internal, and can be created by viruses or parasites or too much stress. These, too, have an energy-draining effect on our bodies. By the time we reach our 40s, many of us have already begun to feel the symptoms of a poisoned system, ranging from chronic fatigue to constipation to sore joints. When this toxicity remains unchecked, far more serious health problems occur as we age.

As the focus of this book is on physical health, this chapter will emphasize toxins that affect our bodies, and offer suggestions to eliminate them. However, it is worth mentioning that one can be *emotionally* and *spiritually* toxic as well. Holding on to anger and resentment can wreak havoc on the body just as surely as a high-sugar diet or nicotine does. With today's economic and social pressures, many of us will find ourselves in jobs and relationships that sap our strength. The disconnection we experience between our bodies and the earth, or between our passions and our heavy responsibilities, can express itself in a kind of listlessness and depression from sources we may not even recognize.

Toxins are a virtually inescapable part of life today, and unfortunately, they are not going away anytime soon. The good news is that we have built-in mechanisms for cleansing, and they are as natural and predictable as the changing seasons. Our bodies will joyfully and capably push out toxins if we have the energy to cleanse and are able to do so regularly.

Before some of the various therapeutic options for cleansing are described, it might help to note a few of the common symptoms of toxicity that you may already be recognizing in yourself.

The Signs of a Toxic Body

Toxins exit our bodies along detoxification pathways. If these pathways are blocked—when our bodies have more toxins trapped inside than can come out—certain symptoms of toxicity will emerge. Here are just a few of them:

- Chronic fatigue
- Headaches
- Arthritis/joint issues
- Hormonal imbalances
- Constipation or diarrhea
- Insomnia
- Breathing issues
- Congestion/runny nose
- Teary eyes
- Nausea

When we remove toxins from our systems, everything begins to work and move around more smoothly.

A good analogy might be when you drain and change the oil in your car. Afterward, your car performs more efficiently and will be less susceptible to breakdowns. This is true of your body as well. With a pure, clean body, all the parts work better. They have greater resiliency and longevity. You manage stress better, you're much happier, and your quality of life greatly improves.

Detoxification Times and Seasons

There are three "seasons" when the body naturally cleanses—spring, summer, and "Indian summer." In the spring, we may notice that we feel achy and that our joints are sore. This is a sign that the liver has gone into a cleansing mode. Summer is also an excellent time for our cells to get rid of impurities, as we tend to be more physically active. The hot weather allows us to eliminate toxins through our sweat glands. We also consume more watery foods that naturally help cool and detoxify. Fresh vegetables and fruits, readily available in this season, aid in the cleansing process.

As fall approaches, the weather turns cold and then, more often than not, suddenly turns warm again for a few more delightfully beautiful days. This is Indian summer; and it can frequently trigger a runny nose, a chest cold, or perhaps even a fever. We often mistake this for disease, but it is nature's way of allowing us one more opportunity to cleanse before we begin to consume more fats and salty foods so that we can be warm and comfortable during the colder winter months ahead. Fats, animal proteins, and mineral-rich salts are warming.

Although your body can push out toxins at any time, it is usually not a good idea to choose to go on an intense detoxification program in the winter. Winter is a time for rest and stillness—a time to accumulate energy, not to cleanse.

With plenty of accumulated energy and with the coming of another spring, new life begins. Spring is a season for renewal, and you can't renew without cleansing. So the cycle begins again.

This cycle of the seasons and the chance to purify is an extraordinary arrangement that we haven't really valued or understood. Honoring nature's laws of cleansing is vital because cleansing is one of our most important tools for staying young.

The body is always cleansing. But when you do decide to aid it in eliminating some of its toxins with a more aggressive cleansing program, it's best to start your cleanse on the days when you're not particularly busy or highly stressed. Many people make Saturday or Sunday their cleansing days, as the weekend tends to be less harried, and there is more time to focus on self-care.

Who Shouldn't Cleanse

Because energy is necessary before we cleanse, there are certain individuals who should not cleanse, either because they need to conserve their energy or because they don't have enough of it to make cleansing viable:

- People who are very weak or recovering from an illness
- People whose immune systems have been compromised or who are critically ill
- People with low blood sugar or diabetes
- People over 70, who must restore energy before they can cleanse
- Pregnant or nursing mothers—it's better to cleanse *before* conception (lower-bowel enemas are fine if constipated)

Cleansing Therapies

Toxicity and detoxification is the number one health concern on many people's minds today. But because we are very busy, we often look for quick fixes—reaching for harsh herbal supplements and laxatives, instead of changing our lifestyles and the way we eat. These quick fixes are often stressful and even harmful to the body. For example, many colon-cleansing products contain strong herbs that deplete the body of important minerals and also drain the adrenals. Many liver-cleansing products have maple syrup, molasses, and honey in them that feed yeast. And the suppositories and chelation therapies (for removing heavy metals) that are available at local health-food stores are a bit like putting the cart before the horse. Most people do not have detoxification pathways that are open enough for these therapies to be effective. These pathways (via organs of elimination) must be strengthened and opened before they will work efficiently.

The Body Ecology program prepares and strengthens the body so that detoxification can occur. The most important way it does this is by promoting foods that create energy and restore digestion. Other therapies help as well.

Foods as Cleansers

By now you have learned quite a lot about the wonderful healing and cleansing properties of food. Below are just a few reminders of why the Body Ecology way of eating is an extremely effective detoxification program.

High-Fiber Vegetables and Grain-like Seeds

Fiber grabs up the toxins and binds them for removal, and it helps reduce constipation. When a stool remains in your colon for too long, the toxins are simply reabsorbed over and over again instead of being eliminated.

Fiber ensures that your food moves through the digestive tract more efficiently, forms a healthier stool, and then leaves your body with ease. It also gives you a feeling of fullness that prevents you from overeating, so it helps with weight loss. In addition, fiber helps regulate your blood sugar by slowing down its absorption rate. When blood sugar is too high or too low, your body becomes acidic (toxic).

Apart from fermented foods, fresh fruits and vegetables are the most cleansing, but fermented foods have the added benefit of assisting with digestion, while raw ones can actually be more difficult to break down (unless pureed, as in a green smoothie). A nice balance of fermented, cooked, and raw vegetables, including sea vegetables, is always best.

Probiotic Foods (Fermented Foods)

Body Ecology has been the leader in promoting fermented foods. Over the years we've received wonderful testimonials about the effectiveness of these foods in helping our bodies become cleaner. The microbiota are powerful scavengers of toxins, including heavy metals.

The good bacteria also kill and suppress the growth of harmful pathogens that produce inflammation and endogenous toxins in your gut. Both pathogens and beneficial microbes can "translocate," but with beneficial microbes as watchdogs, your intestines will contain fewer toxins, and that means that every cell in your body will be healthier. Clean cells live longer, and *you* live longer.

While fermenting young coconut kefir is something new, coconut water has always had a wonderful reputation for helping to cleanse the heart, kidneys, and liver.

Adding a half cup or more of cultured vegetables to your meals gives you another powerful tool for purging toxins. Cultured vegetables, a good fiber source, are usually made with cabbage and may include kale and collards. These veggies are members of the cruciferous family and contain potent, natural antioxidants called *indoles* and *isothiocyanates*. These compounds ramp up your immunity and help protect against cancers of the colon, breast, and respiratory system. Indole-3-carbinol, specifically, protects your cells from damage and hunts down and destroys free radicals; while isothiocyanates are sulfur compounds that have been shown to disrupt the growth and division of cancer cells.

A 4-Day Starter Cleanse

Foods to avoid:

- Animal proteins
- Fats and oils
- Dairy products
- Grains and grain-like seeds

Alkalizing foods to include:

- **Sour fruits** and their **juices**
- **Vegetables**—80% raw, 20% cooked*
- **Ocean vegetables**—rich in minerals
- **Cultured vegetables** and **probiotic liquids**—extremely important
- **Cleansing herbs**—LivAmend helps increase flow of bile from the liver
- **Adaptogenic herbs**—build more energy during your cleanse
- **Water**—add minerals, and drink a gallon per day to flush out toxins
- **Lemon juice in water**—also helps flush out toxins; drink as desired

*Cruciferous vegetables, such as kale and cabbage, should not be eaten raw. Prepare your vegetables in an easy-to-digest format, such as pureed soups and smoothies. These give your detoxification organs a much-needed rest.

The Principles and Cleansing

The Body Ecology way of eating is the ultimate cleansing diet because it quickly strengthens your body and creates more energy. One of its 7 Principles is cleansing. But let's review the other six as they relate to cleansing.

— **The Principle of Uniqueness.** The phenomenon of cleansing is embedded in the very essence of your physical being. Just as you have no control over the rising and setting of the sun, you can't stop your body from pushing out toxins. Some of us are born with a lot more toxins; others have accumulated less. Some of us have more power to cleanse than others. Toxins come out when *they* want to—the best you can do is to help them out. Don't suppress them if you want to grow younger.

— **The Principle of Balance.** Toxins keep us in a constant state of imbalance. Throughout our youth, our bodies make a valiant attempt to stay balanced. At some point they can no longer do so, and those early signs of aging start to show. Actively eliminate toxins and assist your body to achieve balance. Always striving for balance is another phenomenon that was embedded in your body's very creation, but it is always wise to help your own cause.

— **The Principle of Acid/Alkaline.** Toxins keep the body in a constant state of acidity. You already know what that means. Toxic bodily fluids are the perfect environment for fungi, viruses, and even cancer cells to thrive. You want to strive for clean cells that are never too acidic.

— **The Principle of Food Combining.** Undigested food is toxic. Following the food-combining rules creates more efficient digestion and fewer toxins.

— **The Principle of Step by Step.** Incremental steps are particularly important for detoxification, as cleansing should be slow, steady, and deliberate. Cleansing too rapidly can weaken us or even make us ill. Go slowly, but be persistent, never stopping. Cleansing is a lifelong process. The myth that going on a 10-day (or 30-day) cleanse will rid the body of toxins has been circulating around the natural-health community for decades. The assumption is that doing this occasionally is enough. It's just not so.

This principle also helps us better understand the cleansing process. You'll remember that cleansing is related to creating more energy, correcting nutritional deficiencies, and conquering infections.

- **Creating energy:** Because Body Ecology foods quickly strengthen your body, the first thing your cells will want to do is push out toxins. They must do so to live. As you create more energy, you can expect to have moments of joy and occasional moments of discomfort. These ups and downs are all a part of the process of becoming healthy and strong.

- **Correcting nutrient deficiencies:** When you correct deficiencies, your cells come alive again as the missing nutrients work their magic. This creates more energy, giving you even more power to cleanse and create even healthier cells.

- **Conquering infections:** Viruses, fungi, bacteria, and other parasites cause serious endogenous toxins. As your cells and bodily fluids become cleaner, these pathogens won't find you a desirable host.

— **The Principle of 80/20.** Follow these two simple 80/20 rules when you eat:

- **Rule #1:** Do not fill up your stomach completely when you eat a meal. Digestion of food is much more efficient when you leave about 20 percent of your stomach empty. When any food takes too long to break down (or does not do so thoroughly), it becomes another toxin.

- **Rule #2:** At least 80 percent of your meal should be alkaline forming (mostly plant foods), and 20 percent can be acid forming (animal proteins). Too many acid-forming foods are, as their name implies, acidic—and create a toxic environment in your cells.

CHAPTER 19

COLON CLEANSING:
Ancient Detoxification and Hydration Therapy

When we remove toxins from our systems, everything begins to work and move around more smoothly. It is one of the most important ways to stay young.

Colon cleansing has been around for centuries, and is mentioned in Egyptian historical documents as early as 1500 B.C. Russians have long included colon-therapy tools in their spas, recognizing the radiant effect these cleansings have on the skin.

In the U.S., colonics were used quite extensively in the 1920s and '30s, and were considered a common health practice. For the next 70 years or so, their use dramatically declined, along with interest in bowel health in general, and only in recent years has there been a comeback.

Many of the actors and actresses gracing the covers of today's popular magazines don't want us to know that colon-cleansing sessions are their secret tool for remaining young, well hydrated, and healthy. Yes, from beautiful lingerie models to famous opera singers, people find that regular colon-cleansing sessions help with performance and offer wonderful cosmetic benefits. Colon therapy not only keeps our skin glowing and healthy, but it also helps us maintain an ideal body weight. It is now commonly known that the ability to keep off those excess pounds and inches is directly linked to good colon health.

Finally many doctors "in the know" are recommending colonics before a patient undergoes a colonoscopy, in lieu of the highly potent magnesium treatments that can be traumatic to some people.

Safe, painless, and convenient enough to do at home, colon cleansing definitely helps reverse the signs and symptoms of aging. No, you won't find many research studies on colon therapy, but isn't it just common sense? Removing toxic buildup (accumulating inside our intestines for decades) can help revive us and even reverse some of the most serious reasons why we age—inflammation, free radicals, nutrient deficiencies, and cellular debris.

Colon therapy helps correct these issues and also promises improved energy. You will feel more calmer and more focused; sleep better; become more creative; and have a happier, more positive outlook on life. While colon therapy helps reduce the risk of gastrointestinal problems and colon cancer, another important yet little-appreciated benefit is that it is an excellent way to hydrate every cell in your body. And as you know from reading Chapter 12 on hydration, we also age very quickly when we become dehydrated.

Because of its ability to hydrate and then draw out toxins and remove them as they accumulate in your stool, colon hydrotherapy, especially in repeated sessions, actually eliminates toxins from cells everywhere in your body, not just your colon.

Fortunately, colon therapy has become a respected health profession and practice that is undeniably essential due to the increasingly toxic world in which we live. Colonics, enemas, and colema boards offer highly therapeutic interventions.

Not Just for Colon Health— Colon Therapy Is Deep-Cell Cleaning

Colon hydrotherapy is a simple procedure that allows purified, temperature-controlled water to flow slowly into the large intestine, where it gently stimulates the colon's natural peristaltic action to release softened waste. This process is repeated several times in a session and results in better colonic function and elimination. A clean colon is a happier colon.

Clean cells have less inflammation—they live longer, and so will you. Because both disease and health begin in your intestines, you can understand how every cell in every organ and structure in your body—from your brain, lungs, liver, and heart; to your eyes, skin, muscles, and even your bones—benefits from removal of toxic waste from your intestines.

One of the first systems to improve with colonics is your lymph system, which defends your body against infections and the spread of tumors. Lymph nodes (an organized collection of lymph tissue) are numerous in the blood vessels of your intestines and can easily become cancerous when toxic.

Hydrotherapy is an excellent way to remove waste from the small intestine as well. Because the colon and small intestine are connected, when the colon eliminates its material, it signals the small intestine to start eliminating, too.

Emotions and the Colon

Labeling this effective anti-aging tool "colon" therapy downplays its value, because this process also has a profound effect on the emotions. Indeed, your abdominal region houses a very sophisticated nervous system, affectionately termed a "gut brain." This mass of cells in your abdomen is connected to the mass of cells in your skull and to the rest of your central nervous system. It influences the production of neurochemicals, including serotonin and dopamine. When you release toxic material from your gut, toxic emotions (like sadness and anger) leave as well. These emotions are extremely aging, so eliminating them helps you feel more cheerful and serene.

There are basically two types of colon therapy: colonics performed by a professional therapist; and those you do at home with an enema bucket or a colema board (see page 239).

Working with a Professional

If you are new to colon cleansing, you may feel more comfortable with a professional—at least at first. There are two methods available today: the open system and the closed system.

The *open system* delivers a constant, low-pressure stream of water through a small, pencil-sized speculum. You control both the filling and the release of water from your colon with the open system. This method is ideal for those who prefer being left alone in the colonic room, but with a certified therapist nearby to assist as needed. This method offers an ultraviolet filtration system; an odorless vent system; and a sterile, disposable rectal tube. Waste material is flushed away with consistently flowing water but can be seen through a clear view tube. In a *closed system,* the speculum nozzle is closer to the size of the actual rectum, and waste material goes directly into the speculum and from there into a viewing tube. In the closed-system procedure, a certified colon therapist remains in the room with you, controls the instrument, and gives you the colonic. The closed system involves a very thorough release, and the waste material can be viewed and assessed by the therapist.

Anti-Aging on the Cutting Edge

Gently Eliminate with the Luis Rojas Method

While each colon therapist has his or her own unique style, our preferred method at Body Ecology is the Luis Rojas Method. Usually, colon therapists are trained to fill the colon with water and then release all the water and the waste that flows out with it. With the Rojas Method, the colon is slowly and gently infused with filtered water through a small, thin inflow tube until it is well hydrated. When the client feels the need to release, the colon therapist turns a knob on the instrument and the softened waste material is eliminated. Most colon therapists allow all the water to leave the colon after each fill and then once again fill the colon with water. With the Rojas Method, only that single release leaves the body, and then water is immediately introduced into the colon again. This technique keeps the colon filled with water throughout the entire session, and thus well hydrated.

As the colon becomes well hydrated, the older, and perhaps even impacted, waste material inside it also becomes thoroughly soaked, breaks apart, and is more easily eliminated in that session or the next. However, you may be surprised to learn that there is more to the colon-cleansing story. Indeed, done properly with the Rojas Method, you can cleanse toxins from every organ and every cell in your entire body.

Even though we use the term *colon therapy,* the most toxic material in the intestines is stored in the *small intestine.* With the Rojas Method, the years of accumulated material in the small intestine also becomes hydrated and then moves down into the colon, where it, too, is eliminated in future sessions.

The water in the colon cannot go up into the small intestine because of a small valve, called the *ileocecal valve,* which only opens one way. Material in the small intestine can only move into the colon, not the other way around. As I mentioned, the waste material stored in your small intestine is very toxic, and once it begins to appear during your colonic session, your next sessions should be scheduled closer together to remove this material as soon as possible. Not all colon therapists understand this. The material in the small intestine is thick and looks like sludge. It has a very foul odor and contains many parasites, some visible and some microscopic.

We refer to this stage of the therapy as "waking the sleeping dragon." Our bodies adapt and become somewhat accepting of this toxic material, unfortunately, building new cells from it. Now that it has softened up and is ready to come out, you can feel irritable, emotional, and edgy; and symptoms will worsen until you wash it out in your next session.

This material is also preventing nutrients from being assimilated from your small intestine, and removing it will allow you to eat less food but assimilate much more value from the food you eat. This is really the essence of calorie restriction—eat less but assimilate more—one of the most important secrets to preventing aging.

What should you look for in each session? Thanks to the view tube, you can see some of what you are eliminating. Certainly you'll release recently eaten food and older waste material, but much of what you are removing cannot be seen. *Visible toxins,* including parasites (even large colonies of them living in biofilms), *invisible toxins,* including pathogenic bacteria, and *toxic chemicals* (from heavy metals, pesticides, preservatives, and air pollution) are also being removed during each session.

While very few are trained in the Rojas Method (please see sidebar on page 234), you can find a certified colon therapist in your area on the website of the International Association for Colon Hydrotherapy: **www.i-act.org**. Share the Rojas technique with him or her to ensure that you have a much more effective session. (Luis Rojas does trainings in Los Angeles several times a year.)

How Often Should You Cleanse?

A frequently asked question is: "How many colon-cleansing sessions will I need?" Unfortunately, there is no simple answer, as according to the Principle of Uniqueness, each of us is different.

As you begin your cleansing sessions, you will soon be able to judge how many you need. However, cleansing all the cells in your body by working through your colon is not something you do once or twice. Clearing away decades of toxic accumulation is, indeed, a process—one that should continue for as long as you live.

Fortunately, when done properly, colon hydrotherapy is safe, gentle, and effective and will not lead to dependency. In fact, the expansion and contraction of the colon as the water fills and releases will help to tone and strengthen the muscle over time. The hydration is priceless.

When you first begin, you will need to schedule your colon-cleansing sessions more closely together. If done correctly, water from each previous session will also be softening the more stubborn material that may not be released until the next visit. Most colon therapists, naturopaths, and doctors who now recommend colonics suggest you start by having your first six to eight sessions close together.

In future visits, give your colon a chance to recharge—at least one day between each session is best. A professional colonic has more "fills" and "releases" than an enema and can cause your colon to become fatigued if continued for too long on one day. That is why sessions are scheduled for 45 minutes each. With a home enema, you can continue until the water is clear and, if needed, repeat the enema the next day. Questions to ask yourself at the end of the session are: "Did I eliminate well in this session? Should I come back for another right away?"

After Your Colonic

After your colonic, you should go home and take it easy for the rest of the day. Eat a light meal. I do not recommend that you eat raw foods immediately after a colonic. A liquid or pureed soup is best. Probiotic and mineral-rich miso soup is preferred. Eating or drinking probiotics foods (cultured vegetables, young coconut kefir, or a few ounces of InnergyBiotic) is also wise.

You will always benefit from a colon-cleansing session either with a professional or at home when you are experiencing signs of toxicity, such as pain, fatigue, depression, bloating, dry skin and lips, or swelling and puffiness anywhere in your body. If you feel flu-like or if you have the flu, cleansing your colon is a must. You will soon learn to recognize your body's unique way of saying, "I need to eliminate toxins quickly."

Does Colon Cleansing Wash Away Good Bacteria?

Many physicians (who in all truth have usually never experienced colon therapy) have stated that flushing the colon with water depletes it of healthy microbiota. But remember, most microbiota are in the stool anyway and would leave naturally with daily eliminations (if these eliminations are even occurring). Trillions do remain and are not disturbed by the colonic water because they have colonized or settled into healthy mucus.

The fact is, most people are so toxic that when they begin eating the Body Ecology way, they don't have healthy microbes in the intestines anyway. This is why it's so important to eat Body Ecology–recommended foods and liquids, especially probiotics such as young coconut kefir and cultured vegetables. Nutritious and geared toward intestinal health, these powerful foods constantly replenish your colon with a wide variety of hardy beneficial bacteria and good yeast.

Anyone on a high-fiber, sugar-free, probiotic diet like Body Ecology will have excellent colonics. Beneficial microbiota in the fermented foods act like microscopic Roto-Rooters. They are quite masterful at softening the material that has accumulated for years in both your small and large intestines. Imagine millions of microscopic "Pac-Men" working away inside you, helping you to eliminate the effects of improper eating. This is why colon therapists tell us that their Body Ecology clients have the best eliminations during their sessions. Over time, with continual colonics (as needed), years of accumulation in the small intestine will also be cleansed. Your ability to absorb nutrients will increase tremendously, also helping you rejuvenate and live a longer, happier life.

Cleansing at Home

The Home Enema

Only two generations ago, it was common for homes to always have an enema bag. Doctors were even trained in medical school to prescribe an enema when someone fell ill.

An enema flushes out approximately five to ten inches of the lower portion of the colon with water or a special solution. Afterward the person uses the toilet for elimination.

You can find a great deal of information, instructions, and even videos on how to do an enema on the Internet. Enemas have been an important part of our BEDROK (Body Ecology Diet Recovering Our Kids) program for years. Parents of children recovering from autism have found that enemas are very effective at removing toxins, heavy metals, and pathogens quickly—speeding up recovery time.

Enemas are an excellent healing tool for anyone of any age. They are also safe throughout most of a pregnancy. (Stop once the cervix begins to dilate and the mucous plug is released, usually a week or two before the birth.) Breast-feeding mothers will find that their milk is less toxic and even more nutritious when they practice proper colon cleansing with nutritive implants. Find a holistic ob-gyn or naturopath who understands the value of home enemas if you prefer to discuss them with a professional.

One of the benefits of cleansing your colon at home is that you can follow your cleansing enema with a "nutritive implant." Wonderful medicinal herbs and nutrients are combined in a cup or two of liquid (tea or water) and are retained in your colon. This idea is not a new one; practitioners of Ayurvedic medicine have long used these implants, called *bastis*. And they are not new to Western medicine either. In fact, Taber's medical dictionary mentions the use of nutritive implants.

The Colema Board

Cleansing your colon with a colema board is very much like the professional open-system colonic, but can be done at home, where it is private and you can add your own mineral supplements.

To do a colema, you fill a five-gallon bucket with filtered water at body temperature. A strong folding chair faces the toilet. The colema board is placed on the toilet and chair so that you can rest on your back. A pillow and folded towel will make the board comfortable during your colema. The bucket should be placed on a sturdy surface no more than four feet above your colema board. You will then siphon water through the surgical tubing so that it is flowing freely through the rectal tip. Stop the flow of water, lubricate the tip with organic extra-virgin olive or coconut oil, and position your body so that you can insert the tip through your rectum and approximately three inches into your lower colon. Once it's inserted, you can open up the flow of water and begin your colema session.

Setting up and storing the colema board can be an issue if you live in a small space and only have one bathroom. As many of us are now committed to recovering the energy of our youth, I foresee that housing for our aging population will need to change dramatically in the near future. To reflect our passion for rejuvenation, we need smaller homes that require less care but will have wellness amenities that include colonic equipment, a soaking tub, a steam shower and/ or infrared sauna, and a massage table (for in-home visits). We'll also seek homes with plenty of sunlight, a great kitchen for preparation of healing meals, a serene bedroom, lots of thoughtful storage, and definitely a home office. Of course, while we're planning away here, let's not forget that separate suite for our children and grandchildren, who may often visit for their own spa needs as well!

A Note on Colon-Cleansing Herbs and Laxatives

Unfortunately, when people experience constipation or digestive trouble, they often turn to harsh laxatives for relief. Most laxatives—senna, aloe, cascara sagrada, and rhubarb—work by irritating the colon wall so that it will eliminate unnaturally. These should be used sparingly, if at all. Over time, these laxatives can become habit-forming, and the colon will no longer move without their stimulation. They do weaken the adrenals and will continue to deplete your prenatal jing.

For thousands of years, Chinese herbalists created customized formulas for their patients and used a combination of the gentler herbs to stimulate the colon to eliminate. Ayurvedic medicine, which also takes a much gentler approach, uses an ancient herb called *Triphala,* which can be taken every day and is not habit-forming. You may need to take much larger amounts of Triphala at first if you suffer from longtime chronic constipation, and drink plenty of water throughout the day. (*Please note:* Chronic constipation is often caused by low adrenal and thyroid function.)

For better elimination, you can also encourage your liver to produce more bile, which in turn stimulates peristaltic movement in both intestines. (Body Ecology offers an herbal formula with Jerusalem artichoke, sarsaparilla, wasabi, and milk thistle, called LivAmend, which is very effective for this.)

Consistent use of digestive enzymes, especially ones with hydrochloric acid (HCl), pepsin, and pancreatin, also helps improve elimination and stubborn constipation. Of course, eating plenty of fiber and probiotic foods and probiotic supplements (especially a bifidus bacteria supplement) and drinking water so that you are maximally hydrated are musts. (The 80/20 Principle, where 80 percent of your meal is from land, ocean, and cultured vegetables, guarantees an abundance of fiber.)

Herbs and herbal products that stimulate bile or even gentle laxatives like Triphala are best taken *with* meals. They then travel down with the food you eat and help it to move along more effectively. Over time this can help retrain a sluggish colon. But again, chose a gentle herbal colon-cleansing formula and use it short-term.

Even if it seems strange to you, gently infusing water into your colon to hydrate and cleanse the cells throughout your entire body to purify your lymph system, liver, and small intestine should become one of your most valued anti-aging tools. Whether in the hands of a skilled therapist or at home with enemas or a colema board, you will soon learn to recognize how often to use this wonderful tool to help your body become cleaner and turn back the clock.

CHAPTER 20

OTHER CLEANSING THERAPIES:
Useful Additions to
Your Detox Routine

*There are many other detoxifying therapies that can help
enhance longevity, create health, and help us live longer lives.*

Sweating Therapies

In the earlier chapter on cleansing, I spoke of the body's natural
ability to rid itself of waste. One of the principal ways it does so is
through the skin, our largest eliminative organ. According to Mikkel
Aaland, who wrote a book on bathing customs, sweating is essential
not only for detoxification, but as a way to regulate body temperature
and to keep the skin pliant.[1]

Interestingly, the appeal of the sauna surged in the 19th century
after Louis Pasteur's work encouraged more hygienic conditions during surgery and in hospitals. The country that really took the idea and
ran with it was Finland, and the Finns have mastered the art of the
therapeutic sauna. Other cultures have used some form of the sauna
as well, such as the ceremonial sweat lodge of a number of Native
American tribes.

Saunas are a very effective detox therapy. Most environmental
toxins are fat soluble, so they have an affinity for body lipids or fatty
tissue. Metabolic organs such as the liver convert fat-soluble substances into water-soluble chemicals to facilitate excretion. Sauna therapy
can enhance this process by moving these poisons from storage sites

like the liver and putting them "back into circulation," where they can then leave the body through our perspiration.[2] (Colon therapy also helps remove them quickly.)

There are other benefits from saunas! They can restore energy levels, lower blood pressure, improve mental clarity, and enhance liver and immune function.

Anti-Aging on the Cutting Edge

Infrared Saunas

Infrared saunas are a little different from conventional saunas. Rather than turning red-hot, they produce an invisible, gently radiating infrared heat through a ceramic heater. In infrared saunas only 20 percent of the energy is used to heat the air; the rest is used to heat the body. The temperature is adjustable and allows a person to sweat more quickly but also to tolerate longer periods of time inside the sauna.

Infrared saunas are excellent at ridding the body of a wide range of toxins, from heavy metals to other fat-soluble chemicals. They can be an effective treatment for many toxicity-related disorders, such as chronic fatigue, and offer additional health benefits, such as weight loss, improved circulation, pain relief, more vibrant skin, elevation of energy, and reduction of stress. They are excellent for anyone who has sleeping problems. I recommend the Clearlight sauna (**www.HealwithHeat .com**) because it does not emit toxic electromagnetic frequencies (EMFs).

You can also obtain the benefits of infrared-heat therapy in a mat form. The "Biomat" is an FDA-approved medical device that combines therapeutic infrared light, negative ions, and amethyst quartz as a way to reduce inflammation, eliminate toxins, and improve immune-system function. Learn more about it at: **www.biomat101.com**.

Nasal Cleansing—
the Value of the Neti Pot for Eliminating Airborne Toxins

Once viewed as "one of those weird Eastern things," neti pots have entered the mainstream now. They are simply little water pitchers, usually metal or ceramic, used to cleanse the nose, nasal passages, and sinus cavities with salted water. For thousands of years, neti pots have been a basic tool in Ayurvedic medicine, used to wash away dust, pollen, and other kinds of airborne pollution. From the yogis of India to the common man, woman, or child, when we all wake up in the morning, there is an excess of mucus in the upper part of our bodies that needs to be cleansed away.

This type of water cleansing is easy to do and involves tipping your head to the left and pouring water directly into the right nostril so that it flows back out of the left, then switching sides. Use one heaping teaspoon of sea salt to two cups (half liter) of purified water.

Performed daily, just like teeth brushing, cleansing with a neti pot will also improve the health of your eyes, ears, throat, and even your immune system. It is a must if you have allergies, chronic respiratory infections, asthma, or sinus headaches. It reduces sinus congestion and helps prevent colds and flu.

To fight a pathogen or even to prevent exposure to one, you can also add a few drops of antimicrobial essential oil (eucalyptus, tea tree, oregano, or thyme) to the salted water. The water should be close to body temperature—lukewarm-ish. Most health-food stores now carry neti pots that come with instructions for use. Worth owning and using, they're an inexpensive but valuable longevity tool.

Emotional Cleansing

Toxic buildup can occur in our hearts and spirits, just as it does in our physical bodies. By the time we're in our 40s, 50s and 60s, we have stockpiled decades of negative memories, traumas, and unresolved conflicts and resentments. The mind and body are not isolated from one another, but are inextricably linked, and we can see the psychological and emotional origins of many illnesses today. Many of us, particularly those who struggle with chronic anxiety and depression, may benefit from traditional talk therapy with a licensed mental-health-care professional. For others, who may have had limited results in therapy or who are looking for something less time-consuming and costly, there are other helpful methodologies for releasing pent-up emotions and tensions. Many are benefiting from therapies such as Emotional Freedom Technique (EFT) and The LifeLine Technique, developed by Dr. Darren Weissman (see sidebar).

Anti-Aging on the Cutting Edge

The LifeLine Technique™

The LifeLine Technique is an advanced holistic system developed by Dr. Darren Weissman that discovers, interprets, and releases the root cause of physical symptoms and stress. It is a compilation of more than 14 natural-healing modalities—ranging from Applied Kinesiology, acupuncture, and the Five Element Theory of traditional Chinese medicine, to Ayurvedic medicine and the chakras, shamanism, chiropractic, homeopathy, and Neuro-Linguistic Programming—into one seamless system.

The LifeLine Technique facilitates your awakening to the root cause of the painful, scary, or stressful experiences that are manifesting as symptoms, such as physical pain, stress, or anxiety. Until the subconscious is made conscious, we are unable to make a choice or take action based on what we are truly experiencing in any given moment. Coupled with the Five Basics of Optimal Health—the proper quantity, quality, and frequency of water, food, rest, exercise, and owning your power—this technique allows you to create the best possible conditions for the body to heal itself.

Find out more about The LifeLine Technique at:
www.drdarrenweissman.com

Empowering vs. Toxic Relationships

Have you ever spent an afternoon with a friend or relative and returned home feeling worn-out and depressed? It could be that your "friend" is *toxic*. A toxic person is someone who isn't happy until his problems become yours. Are there people in your life who spend a lot of time complaining or blaming others for their troubles? Are you involved with someone who spends all of your time together talking about herself? What about that co-worker who gossips incessantly every time you meet for lunch?

We've all known people who want us to take care of them rather than learn how to take care of themselves. They can sap our energy, and their negativity leaves us feeling helpless and on edge.

We can never entirely avoid toxic people—they are everywhere!—but we can limit the time we spend with them and establish boundaries so that their impact on our emotional lives is slight. Cheryl Richardson, who wrote *Take Time for Your Life*,[3] suggests some questions you might ask yourself about someone you think might be toxic:

- "Am I able to be myself with this person? Do I feel accepted by them?"

- "Are they critical or judgmental of me?"

- "Does the relationship provide an even give-and-take exchange of energy?"

- "Do I feel upbeat and energized when I'm around this person, or depleted and drained?"

- "Does this person share my values? My level of integrity?"

- "Is this person committed to our relationship?"

- "Can this person celebrate my success?"

- "Do I feel good about myself when I'm with this person?"

In short, it is important to connect with people who support us, who celebrate our successes, and who want to give to us as much as to receive. Find these people, and hang on to them! (And encourage them to take better care of themselves, too, so they'll be around for a long time.) They make living joyful and rich.

CHAPTER 21

EXERCISE:
The Gift of Movement

The ability to move with strength, confidence,
and grace is a wonderful gift—and one we become
more appreciative of as we grow older.

Many of us already know how great exercise makes us feel, flooding the body with endorphins and raising serotonin, dopamine, and norepinephrine levels. But more and more research is showing how exercise combats and even reverses many of the degenerative conditions of aging.

An article in *Newsweek* magazine noted the many ways exercise improves brain functioning. Scientists have found that vigorous exercise can cause older nerve cells "to form dense, interconnected webs that make the brain run faster and more efficiently." Aerobic exercise also helps pump more blood to the brain, which means more oxygen to nourish brain cells. Scanning technology reveals that exercise actually causes the frontal lobes to increase in size, challenging the old belief that loss of brain cells as we age is permanent. It has been shown that physically active adults have less inflammation in the brain, so they also have fewer small (and often-unnoticed) strokes that can impair cognition.[1]

But exercise doesn't just affect the brain. Vigorous physical activity has been shown to reduce blood pressure, increase healthy HDL cholesterol, and strengthen cardiovascular capacity. It also increases bone density and size, which helps prevent osteoporosis and sarcopenia (loss of lean muscle mass), two common conditions of aging.[2] Exercise allows your body to modulate blood-sugar levels because it helps create skeletal muscles. Along with your liver, your skeletal muscles help absorb blood sugar, saving your insulin receptors from overload. Without lean muscle mass, blood sugar that is not used by your body is absorbed as fat, which then sends out inflammatory signals, further disrupting insulin receptors. Regular exercise is also a highly effective mental-health therapy, and has been shown to improve sleep, decrease anxiety, and elevate mood.

Getting Started—Exercise Tips

1. **Try to get at least 30 minutes of moderately intense exercise (an activity you can do while breathing harder than normal) a day.** It doesn't work to follow the "weekend warrior" method of cramming an entire week's exercise into Saturday and Sunday. Overzealous weekend exercise often results in injury and undue stress.

2. **Choose forms of fitness that make you happy.** Many of us have mixed feelings about exercise because of how we were introduced to it as children. You may have felt humiliated rather than encouraged, or you might have been alienated by the intense competitiveness of team sports. And the "no pain, no gain" philosophy of many fitness programs makes exercise sound more like an ordeal than a pleasure. If you are coming to exercise later in life and don't know where to begin, you may feel self-conscious about trying something new. Don't despair! Everyone can enjoy some kind of exercise, whether it's walking, biking, Pilates, or ballroom and belly dancing. Experiment and then select those activities that you most enjoy and can excel at.

3. **Set step-by-step, small goals and gradually challenge yourself more.** It can be elating to achieve a health or fitness goal, whether shedding a few pounds or completing a marathon. Listen to your body and follow your own unique pace.

4. Mix it up. It's important to give all of your muscles a workout, with a good blend of cardio, strength, and flexibility exercises. This can be accomplished through cross-training. We die-hard runners might find ourselves struggling with tendonitis and knee issues as we get older. If you're a runner, consider complementing your runs with some core exercises or by taking a Pilates or stretching class for flexibility. If you're an avid golfer, you might consider rounding out your routine with a more cardiovascular-oriented activity such as swimming or biking. As you get in touch with what your mind and body need, you may find that you choose different types of exercise at different periods of your life. Walking, yoga, and t'ai chi are three types of exercise that are excellent for longevity and can be pursued no matter what your age.

Using Exercise to Detoxify

Some kinds of exercise are especially effective at helping you cleanse. For example, it's important to exercise the lymph system when you are detoxifying. It has no pump like your heart, so you must activate it through movement. Daily bouncing on a mini trampoline is the best way to stimulate and move the lymph system. At Body Ecology, we recommend the Bellicon, an excellent-quality rebounder from Germany (**www.QiBounding.com**), but any exercise that results in movement followed by ample hydration and healthy elimination through your intestines (through a normal daily bowel movement or colon therapy) can facilitate cleansing of your lymph system.

Anti-Aging on the Cutting Edge

Becoming Flexible Inside and Out—
Resistance Stretching™

How great would it be if there were one exercise that combined all three fitness objectives—strength, flexibility, and breathwork into one? *Well, there is.* Renowned fitness guru Bob Cooley has developed stretches for 16 muscle groups that use the principle of resistance for improved flexibility and strength. These stretches have immediate and cumulative physiological benefits, along with many psychological benefits. Bob has had incredible results with elite athletes as well as regular folks, and he gathered his ideas into a book called *The Genius of Flexibility: The Smart Way to Stretch and Strengthen the Body.*

To learn more about the Meridian Flexibility System®, go to:
www.meridianstretching.com

5. **Stretch and warm up.** As we age, our muscles get sore faster and stay sore longer. Heating cold and stiff muscles with 15 minutes of warm-up exercises or stretching not only prevents soreness, it also protects us from injury, and allows our muscles to repair themselves more quickly.

So the main takeaway from these past few chapters is this: cleansing is critical to regain the energy of your youth. The wise among us will spend the rest of our lives honoring this important principle.

Over the next few chapters, you will get an in-depth look at ways to restore and increase your energy—methods to bring back your precious prenatal jing.

CHAPTER 22

ENERGY RESTORATION:
Ancient Techniques to Enhance Jing

*Today, the wisdom of the ancients has merged
with ingenious, constantly evolving energy therapies.
Along with pure water, sun, and air, age-defying techniques
make it easy and fun to restore our precious jing.*

By the time we reach our 40s, many of us have strongly ingrained habits that are often harmful. For example, women often get stuck in the "caretaker" mode and feel guilty when they spend money or time on themselves. Many of us, both men and women, have become true workaholics and can't simply just "be here now." Many of us were far more fortunate than our parents and grandparents, and we still have an almost programmed, unquenchable desire to experience and have it all. This has cost us dearly in terms of our precious prenatal jing energy.

Now you've arrived at the time in your life when you *must* start to find therapies to restore that gift given to you at birth. When you begin to search for rejuvenation treatments to increase your life-force energy, you'll quickly discover that there are an overwhelming number of therapies available now, and many more will be emerging in the future. When the choices become confusing, always remember that your time and money are best spent on those that will replenish your prenatal jing. This chapter features a few favorite options pulled from ancient traditions.

So, how does one choose the therapies that are best for your unique brain, body, and spirit?

The Principle of Step by Step is your road map. It teaches that before you can restore your prenatal jing, heal from anything, or even look and feel younger, you must first and foremost create energy. With it, your body will have the vitality to consistently eliminate physical and emotional toxins. With more energy, you will digest your foods better, and your cells will no longer be craving vital nutrients. More energy provides the immune system with the power it needs to overcome fungal, viral, and bacterial infections. And, as each of these causes of aging is overcome, you'll find you once again have more energy. You will be creating a "benevolent" cycle . . . quite the opposite of a vicious cycle that spirals downward, causing you to grow old far sooner than you should.

The Principle of Balance is also about energy. As you practice this universal principle, your goal will be to increase your core energy by creating balance in your body, in the foods you eat, in your relationships, and in the way you structure your time. All of these should be carefully nurtured. Are they making you feel more alive? Or are they draining your inner essence? So it is time right now to begin seeking out those therapies that add more energy, and carefully evaluating those things around you that take away from your constitutional life force.

The Great Healers of Chinese Medicine

No other practitioners of health and healing have focused on creating energy in quite the same way as the great sages of Chinese medicine. For thousands of years, these brilliant healers, who used acupuncture, acupressure, and herbs as natural daily routines, understood that if you "tonify the chi" or create a sufficient amount of energy on a day-to-day basis, your body will take any surplus energy and replenish your prenatal jing while you sleep.

Those of us with more of a Western mind-set might find the concept a little easier to understand if we think in terms of money instead of energy.

Remember your rich "Uncle Freddie" in Chapter 2? He gifted you with $5 million when you were born. Well, let's say that your parents, who were very wise, added to this great inheritance. As you grew up, they taught you to replace any money debited from your account with new deposits as quickly as possible. For example, perhaps you did odd jobs (babysitting or cutting grass or lifeguarding) to make the spending money you needed each week so you didn't have to tap into your inheritance. Even better, you might have often added a little extra to your account knowing that you might need it in the future—to go to college, perhaps, or to buy a house or have a baby. Nevertheless, you didn't touch your precious inheritance unless it was prudent and farsighted to do so.

Now reread the above paragraph and replace money with energy. Your ancestors gifted you with energy. By creating at least enough to use each day, you were careful to never deplete it. At night your body stored what it didn't need. You were mindful to create a way of life where you could often *increase* your energy. At times when you needed to expend extra (to create a baby, or if you were traveling, changing jobs, or moving), you always had enough in your energy account to never deplete your original inherited stores.

Usually, by midlife and beyond many of us become more focused on creating, conserving, and saving money. That's great and usually necessary. However, because of the number of decades we spend literally depleting our constitutional energy, we must now also start accumulating more energy than we spend each day to create a reserve.

It's never too late to start saving and restoring your jing. Whatever you do to replenish your original prenatal energy will enhance the quality of your life. It is also the secret to longevity.

The sun on your skin; the air you breathe; restful sleep; stress-management techniques; the quality of the water you drink; a probiotic-rich, sugar-free diet; the right supplements; and doing exercise that you enjoy will all become important tools to replenish that life-force energy. But can there be anything more? Absolutely yes! Special herbs; fetal sheep cells; stem cells; restoring youthful hormone levels; and even an active, loving sex life can also be powerful tools. So keep reading.

Chinese Herbs for Energy and Longevity

Chinese herbs have always had a prominent place in Asian cultures. They are associated with long life, slowing the aging process, radiant health, physical energy and vitality, mental acuity, and sexual vigor. Entirely natural, these herbs provide special nutrients for physical and mental health, and can be used to treat a variety of conditions, from anxiety to weight problems.

In a conversation with my friend the herbal master George Lamoureux, he gave this advice on restoring prenatal jing:

"In Chinese medicine, there are two organ systems that must be 'tonified' or strengthened as you restore your prenatal jing—your digestive system and your lungs.

"Healthy digestion is crucial for obtaining the nutrients we need from our food, while healthy lungs are crucial for acquiring 'nutrition' from the air. These two energies together create our daily chi—our bodies live and move on them. Create more than enough *daily* chi and you begin to restore your prenatal jing."

Chinese herbs used to increase our day-to-day vitality are *tonic* herbs. Examples of chi tonics are ginseng, American ginseng, white Korean ginseng, cordyceps, codonopsis, and astragalus. Eleutherococcus root is known to increase oxygenation of the blood. When you increase oxygen, it reaches the mitochondria, those microscopic energy factories in each cell, and this increases chi.

Finding that Yin/Yang Balance

In Western medicine it is well understood that the adrenals produce our energy and sexual hormones. Chinese medicine views these organs slightly differently. The kidneys/adrenals are understood to house two separate yet interwoven energies. One is a cooling energy, and the other is warming.

The cooling energy (called *yin/water essence*) controls the fluids in the body, including the saliva; blood; sweat; tears; sexual, lymph, and spinal fluids; and overall moisture. When this adrenal/kidney cooling or yin essence is compromised, you tend to exhibit more sensation for "heat," with depleted body fluids, and dry skin, hair, and eyes. You are most likely often thirsty and become agitated easily and are more inflexible. Three

Sisters is an example of a liquid herbal blend from Jing Herbs (**www .jingherbs.com**) that was created to nurture balance by providing herbs that are cooling and nourish the fluids.

The warming energy (called the *yang/fire essence*) is responsible for sex drive, physical vitality, skeletal structure, willpower, courage, and overall energy. This warming energy enables all organs in your body to function; and when it is depleted, you are lethargic, tired, and introverted. Your immune system will be weak, and you will feel cold all the time. You will be very pale, will have a frail voice, will not have a lot of spark in your personality, and will be more withdrawn in character. Urinary incontinence is a sign of weak adrenals or an adrenal/kidney yang deficiency. For this problem, Jing Herbs created what they call the *Deer Antler Essence.* As you might suspect from the name, it contains deer antler, which is considered very "yang" or strong. To create a balanced formula, two anti-aging herbs, *he shou wu* and *lycium* (goji), were added.

Take a look again at the symptoms you experience when your adrenal/kidney yin and adrenal/kidney yang essences are depleted, described in the two paragraphs above. Add the symptoms together and you have the perfect definition of an aging man or woman. It becomes clear, then, that restoring your adrenals is vital to rejuvenation! (To tonify or strengthen both essences in your adrenals, you would take both formulas.)

Three Brothers is a liquid herbal supplement from Jing Herbs that combines three tonic herbs, each a superstar in its own right. The first of the three herbs is *cordyceps* (a favorite of martial artists and athletes). The second is *astragalus* (a premier herb that increases lung function and builds immunity by increasing white blood cells and natural killer cells). A study at the University of Texas showed that it prevents shortening of the telomeres on the end of DNA strands, greatly lengthening life span. The last is *codonopsis,* which supports digestion and helps keep lungs moist and protected. You could slip several droppers full of Three Brothers into any breakfast drink to wake you up instead of that morning cup of caffeine.

Adaptogens

Most of the tonic herbs are considered adaptogenic. To be called an "adaptogen," an herb must strengthen and provide energy. Examples of some of the most popular adaptogens are panax, Siberian and American ginseng, ashwagandha, shatavari, tribulus, maca, suma, mucuna pruriens, muira puama, rhodiola, schisandra, and matcha green tea.

While adaptogens energize, they also work by calming down negative energy. They help restore your sexual vitality and are excellent for your adrenals. Adaptogens and Chinese herbs work best when combined with the food and lifestyle changes recommended on the Body Ecology anti-aging program.

As we begin to have an even greater appreciation for how valuable adaptogens are for restoring youthful vitality, we'll probably seek out and discover more of them growing all over the Earth—especially in the Amazon rain forest—a potential "Garden of Eden."

My favorite ginseng is Ginex, a white Korean ginseng, grown for four years (not six, as traditional red ginseng is). A simple and very effective way to take Ginex is to add one small packet to a liter of water. Drink this slowly throughout the day. It consistently gives your adrenals and thyroid a shot of energy, which they will love (**www .ginex.net**).

Two other very special herbs worth singling out are holy basil and ashwagandha. Holy basil, also known as tulsi, is not related to the herb basil often used in cooking. It is revered in Tibetan and Indian medicine. It brings down elevated cortisol and sugar levels. It is highly recommended to take one or two capsules from Gaia Herbs if you feel your cortisol levels are too high, especially if you are having trouble falling asleep or staying asleep. Ashwagandha is an Ayurvedic herb that has also been shown to restore prenatal jing energy. To be effective, take 1,500 milligrams in the morning and again at bedtime.

As effective as tonic herbs and adaptogens can be, it is a waste of your money to take them while continuing to eat a high-sugar diet, overindulging in caffeine or alcohol, and failing to manage the stress in your life. Also, please understand that herbs are not substitutes for minerals and vitamins. They do different things in your body.

Stress

We know all about stress, and we tend to take on a lot more of it than we can handle. Because we want to pack as much living as possible into a 24-hour day, we often ignore the toll stress and an overextended lifestyle are taking on our bodies. We forget to take time to decompress and honor our need for quiet and rest.

Stress weakens the immune system, making us more susceptible to a wide range of illnesses, from heart disease to depression. Unmanageable stress often leads to other unhealthy behaviors, such as overeating, drug and alcohol abuse, and destructive relationships.

A little stress is okay. Small amounts can increase the intensity of a good experience and heighten creativity and mental focus. But unmitigated stress—when it persists without the body having a chance to return to its resting state—may be what ages us most quickly. When the famous fight-or-flight response is on overdrive, we start to feel high-strung, irritable, and run-down.

What is happening to us in medical terms? Well, when we find ourselves in a highly demanding situation or an emergency, our bodies are flooded with cortisol, which boosts our immune response. However, cortisol must then inform the immune system that the emergency is over so that it can return to normal. Stress that doesn't die down keeps cortisol circulating in the body for too long, causing our immune cells to become sluggish and opening the door to infection.[1] Interestingly, cortisol also determines where the body will store fat, locating more of it on the belly, rather than on the hips and thighs, where it would be less harmful.

Stress-Management Tips

There are many stress-management techniques, but the most important thing to remember about stress is that we create a lot of it ourselves by trying to be superwoman or superman. Much of our anxiety can be alleviated if we choose to do less and delegate more. When we say, "I don't have time to exercise," or "I don't have time to relax," what we are really saying is "I am not a valuable person unless I am always busy."

Make quiet time for yourself a priority. Actively pursue those activities that support you emotionally and spiritually. This might mean keeping a journal; working on a photo album of your grandchildren; listening to a little Mozart before you go to bed; taking a short, meditative walk in the early morning; or painting a watercolor. Set aside some time each day to do something nice for *you.*

When life becomes too overwhelming, turn to family and friends for support. Even if they can't solve your problems for you, sharing how you feel with an empathetic listener always helps you feel better and arrive at new perspectives and options you might not have been able to come up with on your own.

Massage Therapies

There are many kinds of massage, from Swedish and deep tissue to hot stone and craniosacral. All have a wide range of benefits. Below is a discussion of a special kind of massage called Ohashiatsu®, which is a unique combination of touch and acupuncture.

Ohashiatsu

Developed by a Japanese man named Ohashi who came to the United States in the early 1970s, Ohashiatsu is a special method of touch derived from traditional shiatsu, exercise, and Zen philosophy. Ohashiatsu manipulates the energy within the body, but places an emphasis on the special synergy between giver and receiver. When you receive Ohashiatsu, your posture, mobility, and overall well-being are improved, and it is an excellent way to relieve stress and enhance range of motion. When you give Ohashiatsu, you are energized and rejuvenated by your body's own dance-like movements and the meditative quality of your work. This massage involves deep but pain-less pressure applied to the acupuncture meridians, along with gentle stretches and limb rotations.

To learn more, go to: **www.ohashi.com/ohashiatsu.html**.

Meditation

People practice meditation for any number of reasons—to im-prove concentration and focus, to reduce stress, and even to over-come an addiction. Research reveals that meditation can literally "reshape" the brain and transform the body.

Meditation has been shown to reverse the buildup of plaque in the coronary arteries and to increase antibody levels in the blood-stream, boosting the immune system. It is often used to mitigate and manage pain associated with chronic health problems such as can-cer, high blood pressure, and AIDS. Even more astonishingly, new research is showing that meditation and other relaxation techniques *actually turn off the genes that are associated with inflammation and cell aging.*[2]

Gone are the days when you had to be a mystic to meditate. More and more people are doing it! In 2008, data was released by the National Center for Complementary and Alternative Medicine that showed that 9.4 percent of adults surveyed in 2007 had tried medita-tion at least once during the previous 12 months! Simply sitting in si-lence for 10 to 30 minutes and concentrating on your breath, a word, or an image can clear away the cobwebs and shift the activity in the prefrontal cortex from the right hemisphere to the left, reorienting you from the typical fight-or-flight mode to greater acceptance and equanimity.[3]

Meditation can be divided into two types: *concentrative* and *mind-ful.* In concentrative meditation, you fix your attention on a particular object (a repetitive prayer or mantra), and empty your mind of all other thoughts. As you do this, you try to minimize distractions, con-tinually returning to the chosen object. In mindfulness meditation, you can also focus on your breath or a word or an object, but in this case you keep your focus open. Distractions are not considered intrusions, but rather something to simply observe without judgment or analysis. The emphasis is on staying in the present.

Meditation Practices

There's a meditation practice to suit every need or disposition. Here are just a few of the options out there today:

- **Mindfulness:** Beginning and ending with the breath, mindfulness practice teaches an evenhanded awareness toward whatever thought arises, by simply acknowledging it and returning to the breath.

- **Compassion meditation:** The aim of compassion meditation is outward, designed to foster a feeling of loving-kindness toward a cause or person.

- **Movement meditation:** An example of movement or motion meditation is "walking meditation," which involves walking very slowly, with deliberate and conscious awareness of every step. T'ai chi and qigong might also fall in this category.

- **Transcendental Meditation (TM):** If you're in your 50s, 60s, or 70s, you may remember TM from the 1960s. This type of focused meditation often involves repeating a mantra over and over. Dr. Herbert Benson, author of *The Relaxation Response,* was doing something truly radical in 1967 when he ran various tests on a group of 36 TM practitioners to measure heart rate, blood pressure, and skin and rectal temperatures. He found that when they meditated, they used 17 percent less oxygen, lowered their heart rates by three beats a minute, and increased their theta brain waves (the brain waves that dominate during periods of deep relaxation).[4]

- **Visualization:** This technique involves generating a mental image (a cross, a mandala, a journey, a safe place, or what have you); and can revolve around the achievement of a specific goal, such as losing weight, running a marathon, or curing a disease. This self-aware type of meditation often includes the repetition of an affirmation or intention.

Acupuncture/Acupressure for Rejuvenation

Any discussion of energy would be incomplete without the mention of acupuncture, an ancient Chinese practice (dating to the 2nd century B.C.) used for a variety of physical and psychological issues. Acupuncture and herbs work hand in hand. The herbs can also stimulate the acupuncture points, especially when combined into formulas, but both together is ideal.

Acupuncture utilizes touch and very thin disposable needles to stimulate the body's own healing mechanisms. In a similar way, acupressure uses pressure from the palms, fingers, and thumbs to heal, but without the needles.

The last chapter talked about detoxification pathways in the body that must be unblocked in order for cleansing to occur. We also have energy pathways, called *meridians,* which are routes through which chi energy moves and flows throughout our bodies. Acupuncture points are specific areas along these routes where chi energy collects, which makes them especially significant for healing. These critical points on the body can be accessed through gentle pressure, heat, and more commonly, acupuncture needles.

Anti-Aging on the Cutting Edge

Qigong: Lower Your Blood Pressure with This Time-Honored Energy Practice

We know that stress ages us. It tires us out and weakens the immune system. Eventually, chronic stress will start to show up in our joints and aging skin. This makes qigong, an ancient energy practice from China, an especially effective anti-aging remedy, as it directly impacts our energy and replenishes our blood.

In China, qigong is the name given to the study, practice, and cultivation of *chi,* which we already know to mean "created energy." The word *gong* comes from *gongfu,* which refers to energy and time. Although there are different ways to perform qigong, most practices involve breathing exercises and a series of carefully choreographed movements or gestures designed to facilitate the flow of chi. A consistent qigong practice has the ability to strengthen physical power, increase mental alertness and endurance, and promote long life.

As it relates to longevity, qigong is especially important because, in addition to restoring and moving lost chi, it also replenishes the blood. As we age, our blood supplies dwindle; and our bodies become dry, brittle, and less elastic. In both Western and Chinese medicine, it is our bone marrow that maintains healthy levels of red and white blood cells—the fluid that protects and nourishes the body. Certain qigong exercises restore the suppleness of this marrow, which in turn strengthens the brain and enhances our mental capacity.

In addition, medical studies have found that qigong practice reduces sympathetic activity (the fight-or-flight response that is activated under stress) in the central nervous system. At the same time, qigong increases parasympathetic activity, which is restorative and most active during periods of rest. Qigong is considered a viable therapy for protecting the heart, lowering blood pressure, and reducing anxiety . . . all without the need for drugs![i]

[i]John Seim, "Qigong Reduces Stress in Computer Workers," *Natural News* website, February 25, 2008, **http://www.naturalnews.com/022718.html** (accessed 6/20/11).

Some people have likened chi meridians to a system of pipes through which water flows. The energy in these pipes can get stagnant, impeding or even stopping the easy movement of water. Just as our cleansing pathways must be open and unobstructed, so must our chi pathways be unblocked to allow the free flow of energy. When we are ill, one might say that a pathway has become dammed up somewhere. Acupuncture breaks up the dam.

Shown to increase energy and alleviate pain, acupuncture can also be used to address a variety of other conditions in which the body is in disharmony, such as hormone imbalances; sleep disorders, including insomnia; weight gain; chronic fatigue; anxiety; depression; jet lag; or susceptibility to illness.

The Five Tibetan Rites

The Five Tibetan Rites (also called the Five Rites of Rejuvenation) are another "must-have" in your growing toolbox of anti-aging remedies. Developed by Tibetan monks who condensed 21 yoga poses into 5 yoga movements, these rites were designed to stimulate our energy centers (also called chakras) that correspond to the endocrine glands in our bodies.

The "Rites" were first brought to American readers in a 1939 book entitled *The Eye of Revelation: The Original Five Tibetan Rites of Rejuvenation,* by Peter Kelder, who said he learned them from a wide-traveling retired British army colonel who had lived and studied with Tibetan monks. Subsequent editions of the book have brought these ancient "youthening" rites into the popular mainstream. They are believed to be Tibetan in origin because Tibetan yoga focuses on continuous movement *(Vinyasa)* rather than static poses. Each of the five movements is done 21 times because 21 is a mystical number in Tibet.

The rites lay a good foundation for any yoga practice and should be practiced with a focus on synchronizing the breath. Typically completed in about 15 minutes, the Five Tibetan Rites do not take as much time as a traditional yoga flow series. In a sense, they are the "best of the best."

Anti-Aging on the Cutting Edge

Yoga Nidra

For some of us, it can be nearly impossible to unwind after a stressful day. Our minds race, and our limbs feel restless and jumpy. Yoga Nidra is an ancient practice that means "yogic sleep," and it can be very calming for even the most frustrated insomniacs. When you practice Yoga Nidra, you are brought to a state of conscious deep sleep that is between wakefulness and dreaming. Although you are deeply calm, you are still awake and aware. During Yoga Nidra, the brain is at the delta brain-wave level, which is much slower and is the frequency of deep sleep. An excellent biofeedback practice, Yoga Nidra can involve breathing exercises, body surveys or "scans," and mental points of relaxation. It is ideal for stress reduction, insomnia, asthma, imaginative reveries, and even spiritual explorations.

You can find out more about this unique practice at: **www.holistic online.com/Yoga/yoga_nidra_home.htm**.

The benefits of the Tibetan Rites are many:

- They help detoxify and move the lymph system. (In fact, you may feel a little dizzy when you first start doing them as they move toxins around.)

- They enhance bone mass and help tone your muscles.

- They improve your posture and help create a more flexible spine.

- They flatten your abdomen and help you become more flexible.

- Many report that daily practice soon even eliminates an unattractive symbol of an aging body, the double chin.

A Word of Caution

If you do an Internet search on these exercises, you will discover that there is a lot of variation in how the poses are done and the speed at which they are done. If you are out of shape or unaccustomed to yoga, you might want to do the movements quite slowly at first. Many practitioners report struggling with the poses when they first try them, but then becoming stronger and more adept at them with practice. The important thing is to do them every day. It would be wise for any new practitioner to learn the proper way to do the movements so as to avoid injury. You might try Dr. Dariah Morgan's DVD, which shows the proper way to do the poses and offers modified poses depending on your level of fitness. It offers a warm-up and breathing exercises as well.

The Five Tibetan Rites are described below, with explanations taken from *The Eye of Revelation*.[5] Remember, each one must be done 21 times.

— The **First Rite** (spinning) strengthens the inner ear for balance. "Stand erect with arms outstretched, horizontal with the shoulders. Now spin around until you become slightly dizzy. There is only one caution: you must turn from left to right."

— The **Second Rite** (leg lifts) is for core (abdominal) strength. "Lie on your back full length on rug or bed. Place your hands flat down alongside your hips. Fingers should be kept close together with the finger-tips of each hand turned slightly toward one another. Raise your feet until the legs are straight up. If possible, let your feet extend back a bit over the body toward the head, but do not let the knees bend. Hold this position for a moment or two and then slowly lower the feet to the floor, and for the next several moments allow all of the muscles in the entire body to relax completely. Then perform the Rite all over again."

— The **Third Rite** (camel) activates the spine, opening the heart and solar plexus. "Kneel on a rug or mat with hands at sides, palms flat against the side of legs. Then lean forward as far as possible, bending at the waist, with head well forward—chin on chest. The second position of this Rite is to lean backward as far as possible. Cause your head to move still further backward. Your toes will prevent you from falling over backward. Your hands are always kept against the side of the legs. Next come to an erect (kneeling) position, relax as much as possible for a moment, and perform Rite all over again."

— The **Fourth Rite** (table) stimulates the sacral area and is excellent for building arm, leg, and gluteal strength. "Sit erect on rug or carpet with feet stretched out in front. Your legs must be perfectly straight—back of knees must be well down or close to the rug. Place your hands flat on the rug, fingers together, and the hands pointing outward slightly. Chin should be on chest—head forward.

"Now gently raise your body, at the same time bend your knees so that your legs from the knees down are practically straight up and down. Your arms, too, will also be vertical while your body from shoulders to knees will be horizontal. As your body is raised upward allow the head gently to fall backward so that your head hangs backward as far as possible when your body is fully horizontal. Hold this position for a few moments, return to first position, and RELAX for a few moments before performing the Rite again."

— The **Fifth Rite** (up dog and down dog) focuses on your upper-back muscles and is excellent not only for an immediate elevation in energy but for alleviating stress and depression. "Place your hands on the floor about two feet apart. Then, with your legs stretched out to the rear with your feet also about two feet apart, push your body, and especially your hips, up as far as possible, rising on your toes and hands. At the same time your head should be brought so far down that your chin comes up against your chest. Next, allow your body to come slowly down to a 'sagging' position. Bring your head up, causing it to be drawn as far back as possible."

These ancient traditions are invaluable tools for restoring your prenatal jing. In addition to these lifestyle changes, however, it is important to look at the health of your endocrine system—your hormonal health—to make sure you are nurturing your energy most effectively.

CHAPTER 23

ENDOCRINE HEALTH:
Rejuvenating Therapies

Bottom line: it is essential to evaluate, nourish, and rejuvenate your entire endocrine team—your hypothalamus, pituitary, thyroid, adrenals, and ovaries or testes—to stay young and healthy.

Well over 2,000 years ago, Hippocrates, the father of modern medicine, said, "Let food be thy medicine and medicine be thy food." And yet today, we have come to rely too much on synthetic drugs to cure what ails us. Even advocates of the "natural-foods movement" rely too heavily on vitamin and mineral supplements and components of plants. There are about 60 nutrients known at this time to be essential to human nutrition. Yet even if we swallowed a megavitamin/mineral pill consisting of generous quantities of all these nutrients, we could not maintain our health. This is because whole foods give us something we can't get anywhere else—they contain a live, spiritual essence that modern science has not yet identified.

Supplements can be healthy in the short term, until your inner ecosystem is reestablished. A wise way to supplement is to consider your personal lifestyle and habits. Answer these questions about the supplement:

- Does it create energy?
- Does it help correct digestion?
- Does it help conquer an infection?
- Does it help cleanse toxins from your body?

Remember—toxins are very damaging to the endocrine system. That's why the principles of cleansing set out in Chapter 18 are an important first step in nurturing and healing the endocrine system.

The Adrenal-Thyroid-Pituitary Axis

When I first began studying Chinese medicine, every teacher and book referred to the kidneys as the root of "chi" or life force, supplying energy to all other organs in the body. After many years of relentless personal study, I now believe that this is a modern-day misinterpretation of this ancient system of healing. I believe that what ancient practitioners meant to convey is that *creating energy in a person's body is essential in order to establish, regain, or maintain health.* Certainly your kidneys are important organs, but if it is energy you seek, look to your adrenals.

The Adrenals

While not mentioned in the many textbooks I researched, the adrenals—and the thyroid—are the most important organs of focus if you want to regain youthfulness, health, and vitality. What happens when the adrenals and thyroid have lost their life force or "spirit"? Your digestive system, brain, sexual organs, heart, and central nervous system suffer.

Because of the stressful world we live in, and the confusion and negativity all around us these days, we are often in a fight-or-flight mode whether we realize it or not. This puts incredible stress on our adrenals. We have to find ways to calm them, and then nourish them back to health. In addition to stress-reducing techniques, like meditation and gentle exercise, the following supplements are indispensable to resetting the adrenals. Certain amino acids (GABA, tryptophan, DLPA, and tyrosine), holy-basil extract, B vitamins, and vitamin C help to calm down this fight-or-flight response so that you can then nourish the adrenals back to health. The *shen* herbs, like reishi, help calm the adrenals so that the tonic herbs can start to rebuild them.

Minerals are the most important part of the equation when nourishing your adrenals. Every second of your life, your adrenals must obtain the minerals they need from your bloodstream. How do you ensure that you have mineral-rich blood? An 80 percent plant-based, sugar-free, probiotic diet is a must. A healthy digestive tract that digests food and eliminates efficiently is also essential. While athletes try to replace minerals with sugary drinks like Gatorade, there are far better alternatives. (For more information on mineral supplements, visit: **www.bodyecology.com.**)

Do It Yourself

If you have more time in your schedule, you can make a wonderful soup by slow-cooking organic vegetables and sea vegetables in water for several hours. Discard the vegetables, and you have a mineral-rich vegan broth that you can sip throughout the day. Use this over the course of a few days, or make more and freeze it for later use.

The Thyroid

Then there's the thyroid. Located slightly below the Adam's apple, the thyroid gland is intimately related to our metabolism and how quickly our bodies utilize energy. It helps us make protein, and it controls our sensitivity to the other hormones our bodies manufacture.

To function properly, your thyroid needs zinc, selenium, iodine, tyrosine, and good fats that contain vitamins A and D . . . all of which are found in egg yolks, butter, ghee, red-palm oil, and cod-liver oil. Coconut oil is excellent because it "warms" and "fuels" the thyroid. It also helps speed up metabolism, and can help you lose weight.

The Pituitary and Human Growth Hormone

There's been a lot of talk lately about human growth hormone (HGH), the most abundant hormone produced by the pituitary gland

and the one responsible for the growth of nearly every cell and tissue of the body. HGH affects protein formation, cell differentiation, and cell growth. What most people don't realize is that the pituitary never stops producing growth hormone—even as we age. It simply stops *releasing* it.

Although the impact of this hormone is most profound in the first 15 to 18 years of life, it will continue to influence the deposition of new bone on old bone throughout our lives. For adults, restoring HGH to its optimal youthful level is one of the most powerful of anti-aging therapies, as it causes our cells to regenerate, repair, and replicate.[1]

HGH increases the rate of protein synthesis and the mobilization of fat from fat cells in the body. It also decreases the rate of glucose use. As we age, we release less and less HGH, and by the time we are 60, we only have about 20 percent of the amount we once had in our bodies. Diminishing HGH is called *somatopause,* and it contributes to many of those telltale signs of aging—lower energy and stamina, increased body fat, risk of osteoporosis, decreased sexual function, weight gain, and a greater tendency toward depression and anxiety.

HGH is also essential for hydration. In fact, you cannot correct dehydration in your body if you have low levels of HGH. As it slowly begins to decline, you become more dehydrated and wrinkled. HGH levels also affect your hair color. As the hormone wanes, there is also a gradual dying off of stem cells called *melanocytes* that provide a reservoir for the renewal of pigment-manufacturing cells. Without these pigment-manufacturing cells, your hair becomes gray and loses it shine.

Many people have started taking growth-hormone-replacement-therapy injections, which could have some unpleasant side effects, including swelling of the arms and legs, water retention, high blood pressure, joint pain, and raised insulin levels.[2] These injections are also quite expensive. Ideally, we would begin to generate our own HGH through diet, lifestyle, and important supplements. The high-intensity, short-duration exercise program mentioned later in this chapter increases HGH.

A safer way to increase HGH is to take a secretagogue formula. As its name implies, a *secretagogue* is a substance that causes another substance to be secreted. Amino acids (like arginine, ornithine, lysine, glutamine, glycine, and GABA) and glandulars (usually the hypothalamus and anterior pituitary) are "stacked" or combined, because together they work more efficiently to stimulate the release of your own naturally occurring HGH.

Secretagogues have been on the market for at least a decade. Unfortunately, some of the more effective formulas come in a sachet packet and contain sugar or an artificial sweetener. If you use one of these, be sure to put the ingredients into three to four ounces of young coconut kefir or a probiotic liquid before drinking it. Adding a teaspoon of apple-cider vinegar to this mixture is also wise because HGH naturally depletes potassium, and apple-cider vinegar is an excellent source of this mineral. These tips will help offset some of the negative issues associated with this type of secretagogue.

You can also purchase secretagogue formulas in capsule form and as a homeopathic liquid. These last two do not contain artificial sweeteners or sugar. Because of the recent popularity of secretagogues, more than 75 companies sell them, and there are inferior formulations offered at a low price, so buyer beware.

The anti-aging benefits of taking a secretagogue are all over the Internet. They appear to be true for many and include increased energy and exercise endurance; weight loss; an improvement in skin texture and a reduction of wrinkles; darker, thicker hair; and stronger immunity. Most also report increase in sexual energy, better sleep, and a decrease in frequent nighttime urination.

Secretagogues are not recommended for children, teenagers, or pregnant or lactating women. It is not advisable for diabetics or borderline diabetics to use a secretagogue without the supervision of a physician, preferably one who specializes in anti-aging medicine, because HGH opposes the action of insulin. L-arginine and L-ornithine, two key ingredients in a secretagogue formula, may improve or worsen diabetic conditions. There are no known side effects from taking a *homeopathic* version of HGH.

Hormone Therapy

Many people today reach for the quick fix of hormone-replacement therapy, but when they do, they are not addressing the *real* problem. Typical of our tendency toward narrow thinking, many endocrinologists are prescribing estrogen, progesterone, and perhaps testosterone and DHEA; however, your pituitary and hypothalamus glands are also part of your hormone-producing team. They need your focus and support as well. And of course, don't forget your liver. It *processes* your hormones, so the healthier it is, the healthier your entire endocrine system will be.

If your hormones have started to decline and you are seeing signs of a hormone imbalance, you must begin asking yourself these questions: "Why have I become deficient in these youthening sexual hormones? How can I rejuvenate the organs that produce these hormones so that they'll begin to manufacture them once again?"

Bottom line . . . it is essential to evaluate, nourish, and rejuvenate your *entire* endocrine team—your hypothalamus, pituitary, thyroid, adrenals, and ovaries or testes—in order to restimulate the production of HGH.

Women

Perimenopause can be a very difficult time for a woman today. When her hormones are out of balance, she'll feel quite unhinged until she finds her way to a savvy endocrinologist experienced in *bioidentical* hormone-replacement therapy. Most women believe that a decline in estrogen and progesterone is an inevitable part of menopause. But with proper diet and supplementation, it is possible to have healthy ovaries and adrenals (the two organs that produce most of your estrogen and progesterone) even if you have entered perimenopause or menopause.

Although a woman may benefit from testing and individualized hormone supplementation, the fact is that our hormones are always fluctuating throughout the day. Even bioidentical hormones, while a dramatic improvement over synthetic hormones, can never exactly mimic the fluctuations and rhythms of our own naturally produced hormones.

Testing your hormones at least twice a year is wise. However, you might consider postponing your next set of tests until *after* you've been on the Body Ecology program for several months. Many women find that their hormones balance out significantly and that they no longer require hormone treatments, or they only need minimal amounts.

As a woman, you should know that when your estrogen levels drop, you will most likely suffer from low levels of two important, feel-good brain chemicals—serotonin and dopamine. These brain chemicals are very much related to mood and happiness.

Because low serotonin causes both depression and low self-esteem, you can see how this might negatively affect your relationships. Bad relationships seriously drain a woman's energy. Both stress and a diet of excessive animal protein are especially harmful for a woman, because they lower serotonin. A woman needs to feel calm and needs to eat much less animal protein than a man. Seasonal affective disorder (SAD), or a lack of exposure to sunlight, especially in the winter, also depresses serotonin levels.

With low serotonin levels you will find yourself craving carbohydrate-rich foods. You may have all the willpower in the world, but there is a true biological reason for your cravings for chocolate. Your brain is always trying to achieve balance and when stressed, wants to feel calm again. It's no surprise that chocolate is a favorite food of many women, as it increases endorphins and temporarily elevates both dopamine and serotonin. But chocolate is very high in oxalates, makes you more acidic, and is usually combined with sugar. Both chocolate and sugar are addictive and age you quickly.

Drugs that increase serotonin levels are not the answer. Low serotonin levels cause constipation, and while these "serotonin reuptake inhibitors" may temporarily relieve you of constipation, they soon *cause* it again as serotonin levels increase and then become too high. Healthier choices are the supplements 5HTP and tryptophan, an amino acid. Either can be taken in the morning or at bedtime to increase serotonin levels naturally. Serotonin Luxe is one of our favorite products for increasing serotonin naturally (visit **www.bodyecology** **.com**).

While women have less dopamine in their brains than men do, you won't feel content or at peace with life when your levels of this neurotransmitter are low. Declining levels of dopamine can lead to restless legs syndrome, fibromyalgia, or Parkinson's-like symptoms. In midlife, this combination of declining estrogen and dopamine may create mood swings, severe hot flashes, night sweats, or sleep disturbances.

Fortunately, the amino-acid supplement tyrosine can help normalize dopamine levels in your brain. If you have cancer, do not take tyrosine, because certain types of cancer use amino acids to fuel their growth. If you are on an antidepressant medication, you should only take tyrosine under your doctor's supervision. Tyrosine affects mood, and you may need to adjust your dosage, but we recommend 500 milligrams in the mornings as a start. It's great for your thyroid and the prefrontal cortex of your brain, too. Take tyrosine in the mornings, as it can keep you up at night if you take it close to bedtime.

Mucuna pruriens, an ancient herb from India, also increases dopamine levels in the brain and can be taken at any time of the day. PEA (phenylalanine), the chemical found in chocolate and cocoa, increases dopamine as well. E_3Live, blue-green algae from Klamath Lake, is rich in PEA.

Clearly, because of the close connection between your hormones and your brain chemicals, it would be wise to have your doctor test your amino-acid levels to see what brain chemicals you may be deficient in.

Relationship expert John Gray, Ph.D., has written a fascinating book about our hormones and brain chemicals. It is an enjoyable read for both men and women who want to better understand their emotions and behaviors and those of others. Dr. Gray's book is called *Venus on Fire, Mars on Ice: Hormonal Balance—the Key to Life, Love, and Energy.*

Men

We sometimes forget that men also have their hormone challenges. Men should have their HGH, DHEA, estrogen, and testosterone levels checked twice a year. In men, the hormone decline of testosterone in particular can be subtle and incremental, while estrogen levels can climb too high. They may find that they aren't as self-confident or as motivated as they used to be, or may even struggle with depression or sadness. One day they wake up and find they're in the throes of the "grumpy old man" syndrome.

Acupuncture is an excellent therapy for balancing hormones in men, and Chinese tonic herbs, mentioned in the previous chapter, help restore energy to the adrenal/kidney meridian in the body. Walking or other daily exercising is a must to keep levels of hormones like DHEA and HGH high, but even with exercise, it may be necessary to use a small amount of all the natural, *bioidentical* hormones that you are deficient in.

Don't underestimate the importance of testosterone. It isn't just for sex drive and sperm count. It also helps maintain bone density, muscle mass, and red-blood-cell production. For most men, a more noticeable decline in testosterone starts in the mid-40s, and so does this common yet unnecessary symptom of aging: a decrease in muscle mass, with an increase in body fat. Unfortunately, reduced physical energy and endurance, gradually decreasing libido, loss of bone density, and an increase in cholesterol accompany this decline in testosterone. A deficiency of testosterone has even been cited as a precursor to cancer. Search for a physician trained in functional medicine with a specialty in hormone and anti-aging therapies. (Go to **A4M .com** for a referral.)

Dopamine is a brain chemical that is vital for a man's happiness, and it, too, decreases with age. Lower levels intensify the negative effects of low testosterone mentioned above. Anxiety, depression, cravings, and addictions all can be traced to low levels of dopamine. This neurotransmitter helps keep us alert, active, and motivated. Sexual desire and feelings of excitement and pleasure decline as dopamine declines. General symptoms of aging such as poor sleep; fatigue;

depression; decreased muscle tone; and loss of cognitive functions, like memory, alertness, concentration, and decision-making, can become issues. A man with low dopamine levels loses his ability to make executive decisions.

Dopamine has a positive effect on heart and circulation. It keeps a man's metabolic rate high. As his metabolic rate declines, he puts on weight. Dopamine is essential for control of movement. Numerous research studies have identified low levels of dopamine as a cause of Parkinson's disease. As mentioned previously, tyrosine, mucuna pruriens, and PEA from E_3Live Klamath Lake blue-green algae help increase dopamine.

While today we have the luxury of bioidentical hormones and natural supplements that increase neurotransmitters such as dopamine and serotonin, bioidentical hormones will soon be seen as merely a temporary bridge to something even better. With new inroads in stem-cell therapy, we will soon be able to produce these hormones again on our own.

Stem-Cell Therapy

There are few areas of medical science that are more fascinating and have as much potential for transforming how we think about healing, longevity, and quality of life than stem-cell research.

Whether used preventively or as an active intervention, stem cells are the latest anti-aging miracle. Found in almost all multicellular organisms, they are unique in that they not only have the capacity to renew themselves, but they are also able to *differentiate*—to develop into specialized cells that make up a variety of our organs and other tissues. They can literally transform themselves into any other type of cell in the body, which is why they have been called the "building blocks of nature," with potential to treat numerous diseases and traumatic injuries, as well as to regenerate entire organs.

You may not be aware of this, but you've been using stem cells your entire life. Think of them as the body's MASH unit—they see trauma and quickly mobilize to fix it. When you cut your finger or get a sunburn, stem cells receive the alarm signal and rush in to repair the damage.

There are two basic kinds of stem cells—those found in most adult tissues and those found in the cells of three- to five-day-old embryos. Adult stem cells, found in brain, bone marrow, muscle, skin, blood, liver tissues, and especially adipose (fat) tissue, can change into most cell types.

The stem cells found in three- to five-day-old embryos (embryonic stem cells), on the other hand, are pluripotent—that is, they have the unique ability to develop into any of the 220 cell types in the human body.[3] But it's not just embryonic stem cells that have this ability—umbilical-cord and placental stem cells are also pluripotent. In fact, researchers have found strikingly similar characteristics between cells taken from the outer membranes of the amniotic sac and embryonic stem cells.

Bone-marrow transplant, a stem-cell therapy that has been used for many years as a treatment for leukemia and other types of cancer, is well known today. But as mentioned above, stem cells can also be derived from umbilical-cord blood and the placenta, as well as from the Wharton's jelly in the lining of the umbilical cord, from peripheral blood, and even from menstrual blood.

But what does all this have to do with aging?

Stem-Cell Therapeutics and Aging

The first implication of stem cells for aging should be obvious. When organs fail or wear out over time, stem cells may have the capacity to bring them back to life again. In this sense, they might be used to restore our prenatal energy, to grow new teeth, replace exhausted livers and kidneys, and repair damaged limbs. Imagine if our adrenals and glands such as the hypothalamus, pituitary, and pineal thyroid could be reenergized with stem cells? Phase III trials in the U.S. are revealing how stem-cell products might address a range of indications, including osteoarthritis, Alzheimer's, heart disease, Crohn's, and Parkinson's, particularly when treated in the early stages. Furthermore, in Panama there have been several cases in which spinal-cord injuries were reversed; and numerous cases of multiple sclerosis, rheumatoid arthritis, and autism markedly improving using both allogenic (donor) umbilical-cord cells and autologous (native) bone marrow– and adipose-derived stem cells.

And there are cosmetic impacts as well—for example, *mesenchymal* stem cells, which are particularly effective at rebuilding tissue, bolstering immunity, and combatting inflammation, have been used as anti-aging treatments, offering patients noted improvements in restoring hair to its original color, creating a smoother complexion, and reducing age-related pigmentation marks.[4]

Scientists have recently found a type of stem cell in hair follicles that is capable of making epidermis, sebaceous tissue, and more hair follicles—in short, new skin and hair. Paul Sanberg, professor of neurosurgery and director of the University of South Florida Center of Excellence for Aging and Brain Repair, points out the profound implications this could have for cosmetic skin repair and grafting, and perhaps even for hair replacement.[5]

But there's a second, possibly more important thing to understand about stem cells. Research and early clinical studies have proved that stem cells can release nutritional or "trophic" factors that can be of great benefit. At the University of Buffalo in New York, mesenchymal stem cells (MSCs) were injected into hamster leg skeletal muscles. Not only did the MSCs not migrate away from the target area, but they also released trophic factors that traveled to and repaired the severely damaged heart.

What's more, just injecting the trophic factors without the cells into leg skeletal muscle had about the same benefit as the cells had! This has huge clinical implications . . . think how wonderful it would be to treat heart disease and many other conditions with either intramuscular shots of MSCs or even just the trophic factors. For those interested in learning more, please see the free online article entitled "Heart failure therapy mediated by the trophic activities of bone-marrow mesenchymal stem cells: a noninvasive therapeutic regimen" (available at: **www.ncbi.nlm.nih.gov/pmc/articles/PMC2716100**).

As we get older, our stem-cell reserves decline, we aren't able to produce new ones, and the ones that we have become less robust. But scientists are discovering that the environment in which these cells exist also matters. If that environment is inflamed, it can impede the functionality of stem cells—they can no longer do what they are intended to do.

A study conducted at the University of South Florida has found that the injection of human umbilical-cord cells can assist an aging brain. When umbilical-cord blood cells (UCBCs) were injected into aged laboratory animals, improvements were found in the microenvironment of the hippocampus (an area of the brain that plays an important role in long-term memory and spatial navigation), and there was also a measurable rejuvenation of the neural stem/progenitor cells.

"Brain cell neurogenesis (new cell development) decreases dramatically with increasing age, mostly because of a growing impoverishment in the brain's microenvironment," says study co-author Alison Willing, Ph.D., of the Center of Excellence for Aging and Brain Repair. According to researchers, the decrease in neurogenesis that accompanies aging is a result of a decrease in proliferation of new stem cells, not the loss of existing cells. However, the improvements they saw did not come from direct replacement of cells but by changing the microenvironment of the brain in which the cells reside. Willing added: "The increase in neurogenesis we saw after injecting UCBCs seemed to be due to a decrease in inflammation."[6]

Once again we see the enormous role that inflammation plays in aging. Do you remember the factors that cause inflammation? Food with pesticides, environmental pollutants, mercury in the air we breathe, excess body fat, poor diet, lack of exercise, and even genetic predisposition can contribute to inflammation in the body. As we age and become more inflamed, our brains shrink, and the stem cells that might be on the ready to repair them just aren't functioning as well anymore.

In fact, any of the above can contribute to neurotoxicity, and can lead to disabling genetic defects in the neural stem cells. Research in mice has shown a 2-month-old mouse will have about twice as many neural stem cells as a 24-month-old mouse. This loss in brain stem cells is likely tied to most all neurodegeneration that occurs with advanced aging, or even earlier if there is enough neurotoxicity present.[7]

The implications of this should be obvious. People who live a healthy lifestyle have lower inflammatory markers—markers that prevent healthy stem cells from being released. Lifestyle can turn down the "hot-water faucets" of inflammation inside us and create the kind of healthy environment we need to get those stem cells activated.

If you eat well, sleep deeply, exercise regularly, are well hydrated, and have high/normal vitamin D levels, many more stem cells will be released from your bone marrow and you will age slowly. With this new understanding of stem cells, medical textbooks will now have to be rewritten to say that in many ways, death and aging are a sign of insufficient stem-cell production in your bone marrow. Viruses and toxins from heavy metals, pesticides, and chemicals cause mitochondrial failure in your bone-marrow cells so that they cannot produce healthy stem cells.

Exercise Mobilizes Stem Cells

It's especially important to note that exercise is one of the primary ways we can create new stem cells. When we exercise, there are six to eight times as many stem cells present in our peripheral blood. Here's an example of what exercise can do for one area of the body in which we often see signs of aging—our brains.

As we age, our cortisol levels increase, and the hippocampus decreases in size. The hippocampus, as noted before, is related to memory and plays a big role in dementia. Exercise can help the hippocampus to regenerate. A stem cell will re-create the cell that is needed, in this case a neural cell, and at the same time it will replicate itself. Working with aged mice, researchers in Florida have demonstrated that a single injection of human umbilical cord blood mononuclear cells (HUCBMCs) can rejuvenate a mouse's hippocampus and supply of neural stem-cell progenitors. The aged mouse brains also began producing new nerves. And this type of therapy doesn't have to be invasive. It can be introduced into the peripheral veins (injected in the arm) rather than directly into the brain.[8]

So, basically we've added a new theory of aging—the *stem-cell theory*. We age because we stop releasing adequate numbers of stem cells. What we eat, how we think, the people we surround ourselves with, and how many toxins we are storing in our bodies all impede the activation of these cells. Rejuvenation begins with the reactivation of weaker, dying cells first, followed by the restoration of new stem cells that have been lost.

Other studies have shown that the optimal conditions for stem-cell release are related to being properly rested—this means that sleeping regularly and restoratively, managing our stress, and finding balance in our lives can affect the maximal release of stem cells. Paul S. Frenette, M.D., professor in the Department of Medicine at Mount Sinai School of Medicine, writes: "We don't know why stem cells circulate in the blood but the maximal release of stem cells in the circulation occurs when the animal is resting. This argues for a role in regeneration."[9]

One of the most exciting uses of stem cells has been the regeneration of tissues. Anthony Atala, M.D., the head of the regeneration program at Wake Forest University, stated that his researchers have grown nearly two dozen different types of body parts, including muscle, bone, and a working heart valve. He went on to say: "I think if we start combining things like better prevention, better care, doing things better for our body, and just with regenerative medicine, we may push [our life spans] up to 120, 130 years."[10]

New Discoveries on the Stem-Cell Frontier

Dr. Leonard Smith, medical advisor for this book, is a volunteer on the surgical staff at the University of Miami, and medical advisor for the University of Miami Department of Integrative Medicine. He is also a consultant for the Institute for Cellular Medicine, which specializes in research and clinical stem-cell therapy, and publishes articles on stem cells in peer-reviewed journals. Located in Panama City, Panama, the Institute has treated more than a thousand patients.

When researchers at the Institute began their work several years ago, they worked solely with umbilical-cord stem cells. Today, they also use bone-marrow cells and fat-derived stem cells from liposuction, with good results, especially in the area of autoimmune diseases. Promising outcomes have also been seen for autistic children and people suffering from multiple sclerosis, renal and heart failure, rheumatoid arthritis, and osteoarthritis. In addition, they have treated several paraplegics with spinal-cord injuries who are now recovering nicely, including walking again.

Now affiliated with several universities, the work done at the Institute may be on the cutting edge of stem-cell advances. (For more information on the Institute for Cellular Medicine, go to: **www.cell-medicine.com**.) There are increasing numbers of stem-cell clinical trials now taking place in the U.S., mostly at universities. There are, however, some publicly traded companies doing stem-cell trials. Ongoing clinical trials on type 1 autoimmune diabetes are under way all over the world. Just like computers changed the world we live in forever, it is becoming quite obvious that stem-cell therapy has the potential to benefit humankind in many ways that were unimaginable to out ancestors.

Classic Cell Therapy

Stem-cell therapy has marvelous potential for the treatment of our most feared illnesses, but it is primarily aimed at a single disease process or traumatic injury. There is another kind of cell therapy that offers anti-aging benefits. It complements stem-cell therapy because it doesn't just treat a single organ or gland, but reaches into *all* organs, endocrine glands, and connective tissues. We call this more comprehensive kind of cell rejuvenation "classic cell therapy" to differentiate it from stem-cell therapy.

Classic cell therapy was introduced by Dr. Paul Niehans of Montreux, Switzerland, in 1931, when he injected calf parathyroid into a patient whose parathyroid glands had been damaged during thyroid surgery. The patient survived and went on to live a healthy life into her 90s. Variations of this method have been practiced in the 80 years since then, and during his lifetime, Dr. Niehans went on to treat many heads of state and movie stars of the World War II era and beyond. Mick Jagger uses this type of therapy, as did Dick Clark, to stay remarkably energetic and to look much younger.

The goal of classic cell therapy is to slow, and even reverse, biological aging. The focus is on the immune and endocrine systems, as well as connective tissue. Breakdown in these areas is the cause of aging and is responsible for most chronic disease.

The cells used in classic cell therapy are slightly more mature than stem cells, resulting in an organ-specific cellular serum. The tremendous advantage to this is that the cellular serum can be administered intramuscularly and will migrate to the target organ—that is, heart to heart, lung to lung, and so forth. This has been demonstrated by radioisotope tracing studies.

Further studies at the Pathological Institute of the University of Munich have shown that protein biosynthesis in the targeted organ will increase by up to 100 percent compared to untreated organs, resulting in renewed vitality and function, commensurate with a younger biological age.

My good friend Judi Smith, with the International Clinic of Biological Regeneration, has developed a protocol reflecting more than 30 years of experience in the field and major pharmaceutical advancements. This protocol is designed to treat the body as a whole, and then to target specific organs/glands relating to immune and endocrine function, the connective tissue, and skin, as well as the pituitary, hypothalamus, and adrenal glands, to support immune function and reduce inflammation. Other serum preparations can be customized to address the specific concerns of each individual. This combination, particularly when administered periodically (three to six months apart), can have significant positive impact on both appearance and vitality.

The idea is not just to look and feel as great as you can, as long as you can, but to also have the vital energy to pursue your interests and passions. While classic cell therapy can't prevent aging entirely, it can slow it down considerably and even give you more energy like you had when were much younger. And now, of course, you hold a "bible" in your hands that provides you with all you must do to actually reverse the "hands of time."

Our knowledge of stem-cell, trophic, and gene therapy is evolving at a tremendous speed. With new insights being reported every day, this is an exciting time to be alive—for every generation.

Healthy Sexuality—Doing It Without Drugs

For many people "life after 40" includes more satisfying and meaningful sexual relationships. The urgent hormonal drives we experienced when we were younger will have abated a bit, and most of us are no longer focused on conception and starting a family. But these changes in lifestyle and drive don't mean we no longer want, or can't have, fulfilling intimate relationships. In fact, with more of us single today than at any other time, we are more willing to enjoy our sexuality and meet each other in nontraditional ways, such as online social-media sites. And because women of this generation tend to be more educated, career-oriented, and affluent, they aren't necessarily dating in order to "settle down" and get married. They view their sexual relationships as just one more aspect of a fulfilling life.

It should be noted, however, that many of us who came of age before the HIV epidemic don't have a sense of the dangers of sex that younger generations do. Women over 50 are at risk of developing HIV from heterosexual sex because their thinner vaginal walls are more susceptible to cuts and tears. The number of new HIV infections among older women is rising, and AIDS cases among women 50 and older nearly doubled between 1988 and 2000.[11]

And what about sexual-performance issues, particularly in men, whose problems with erectile dysfunction dramatically increase with age? Too often, we want a "quick fix" approach to sexual problems or waning sexual energy. If something isn't working, or isn't working as it did when we were 18, we reach for a pill. But magic pills like

Viagra and Levitra don't address the underlying conditions that may be producing sexual dysfunction, and for many, they simply don't work at all.

Al Sears, a Fort Lauderdale physician, has developed a 12-minute exercise program called PACE, which advocates shorter bursts of intense exertion as a healthier means of losing weight and staying fit. It has the added benefit of improving one's sexual performance. Short bursts of vigorous exercise cause an increase in blood flow and boost the supply of nitric oxide in the body. Being able to release nitric oxide is critical to erection of the male penis and female clitoris for sexual responsiveness. Our supply of nitric oxide declines as we age, and this is one reason why older men and women often report declining performance in the bedroom.

High-intensity workouts are a great way of improving nitric-oxide production, but as we grow older this can be more challenging, as we have less stamina during rigorous exercise. Sears recommends a more incrementally intensive program that allows exercisers to control and manage their own progression.

Sears's PACE program increases endorphins—those feel-good chemicals in the body—as well as brain chemicals like serotonin and dopamine, which make us feel content yet excited about life. Peri- and postmenopausal women, in particular, can be quite low in endorphins and brain chemicals because these decline as estrogen declines. HGH and testosterone levels also increase dramatically when we exercise.

The PACE program is a form of interval training that uses running as the mode of exercise. This is fine, but for many people over age 40, running may be too stressful on the joints, ligaments, and tendons. Rapid walking may be more appropriate and is just as effective. Interval training with swimming, with elliptical cross-training machines, and even with weights can be done. *The key is to exercise at maximum or near maximum intensity for 10 to 60 seconds and then rest or go slower for 30 seconds to two minutes, and then go fast again.* Interval training increases the release of growth hormone, insulin-like growth factor one (IGF-1), and testosterone; and helps lower blood sugar and sensitize insulin receptors. All of these are critical for optimal sexual performance for both men and women.

In addition, this program increases the intake of oxygen by increasing the capacity of our lungs and preventing them from shrinking with age. This in turn ensures that our energy levels rise; excess fat is burned; and the anti-aging process is activated by the dynamic regeneration of cells and tissues inside the body, including increasing the number and function of mitochondria, our energy producers.

Anti-Aging on the Cutting Edge

Tantric Sex

Many people have misguided notions about tantric sex, assuming it must involve never-before-discovered erogenous zones, techniques, and positions. Basically, tantric sex is "What's the hurry?" sex. For most people, the typical sexual experience lasts approximately 15 minutes, yet most women take at least 20 minutes to climax. What's wrong with this picture? Tantric sex is *sensual sex,* intimacy that focuses on extending the sexual experience and satisfying your partner on a spiritual and emotional level, as well as on a physical one.

Like most exercise, interval training will also decrease total body inflammation as long as you don't overdo it. Remember to start slowly, then gradually increase the intensity and decrease the amount of time in between each exercise.

Here is a PACE outdoor-running workout proposed by Dr. Sears.[12] You can do this walking as well.

1. **Warm up.** Warm up for about one or two minutes.

2. **Start.** Once you're warmed up, start at low to moderate intensity, and increase the level of intensity after each set. Start first by running (or walking rapidly) for two minutes.

3. **Recover.** Now relax. Notice your heartbeat, and keep track of how long it takes to get back to normal.

4. **Repeat.** Then run for 90 seconds, followed by rest. Repeat this; and decrease the exertion period each time from 90 seconds to 45 to 30 and then to 20 seconds for a total of six sets. This shouldn't take more than eight to ten minutes.

Anti-Aging on the Cutting Edge

Whole-Body Vibration:
A Way to Enjoy the Benefits of Exercise

When you hear the words *vibration machine,* you might get a mental image of an overweight woman wearing a wildly vibrating belt that shakes and bounces the cellulite from her hips. Fortunately, we've come a long way from those funny contraptions of the 1950s! In fact, vibration technology is said to be the medicine of the future and the ideal anti-aging tool. I own a machine and love it.

The first generation of whole-body vibration machines appeared on the market in the '70s, and today there are more than 30 different companies making them, ranging in price from $700 to $15,000. They can be found in the homes of professional athletes, dancers, entertainers, physical therapists, doctors, and authors. However, it pays to do your homework before purchasing one.

How Whole-Body Vibration Works

With most whole-body vibration machines, you stand on a platform that vibrates rapidly with a motor that creates either a vertical, a vertical and horizontal, or a seesaw movement. On the motor-driven machines, you stand on a platform and do workout sessions and resistance-training exercises. This produces very effective results in a shorter time than without the machine. While motor-driven machines are mostly for exercise, they do cleanse your lymph system and stimulate circulation. A professional trainer will give you the best results and customize workouts for your unique body type, changing them as needed. All machines come with educational materials that demonstrate how to use the equipment in your home.

Motor vs. Sound-Wave Vibration

The safest and most medicinal whole-body vibration machines use sound waves under the platform to create a vertical vibration that can be adjusted, offering a wider range of vibrational frequencies and medicinal benefits. You can stand or sit on these machines and can practice qigong or meditate. If you have a weaker constitution or an injury, or are struggling with osteoporosis, this is the vibration machine for you. The motor-driven ones can be injurious to hips and knees, while the sound-vibration ones are softer and gentler—perfect if you have physical limitations. And if you just won't exercise because you lack the time or desire, sound-vibration machines provide many of the benefits of exercising without the exercising.

My own sound-wave vibration machine—the TurboSonic X5—stands proudly in my home (**www.turbosonicusa.com**). I also highly recommend the new SonicLife (**www.soniclife.com**), a less expensive version of the TurboSonic, but just as effective.

The Benefits of Whole-Body Sound Vibration

In addition to feeling and looking vibrant when you step off of a sound-vibration machine, you will immediately notice improvements in balance, a common problem as we age. The gentle vibration stimulates the middle ear so your sense of equilibrium improves; while you also build muscle, tendon, and ligament strength. But there are many other benefits:

- Cleanses the lymph system and stimulates circulation
- Improves blood pressure, digestion, sleep, stress, and overall mood
- Stimulates healthier, more resilient cells
- Creates stronger, better-defined muscles
- Lowers cortisol and naturally increases bone density, testosterone, and growth hormone
- Promotes cellular waste removal, increasing your ability to detoxify

Exercise is just one way to bolster healthy sexuality. Dr. Ridwan Shabsigh, a certified urologist specializing in sexual health, encourages people to see their sex lives in the context of better overall health.

He points to the conditions that can contribute to sexual dysfunction—from diabetes and obesity; to cardiovascular disease, depression, and drug and alcohol abuse. Dr. Shabsigh's holistic approach looks at overall lifestyle choices—diet, exercise, supplements, stress reduction, avoidance of self-destructive behaviors, and commitment to a partner—and how these issues can positively or negatively affect sexual function.[13]

There's no reason why sex can't be "sensational" as we age, argues Shabsigh, and for many, sexual intimacy is better than ever before because we've learned and grown wiser from past relationships. We are much more in tune with our bodies now, and we are, in turn, more attuned and attentive to the needs of our partners.

As the years come and go, you may no longer have the sexual motivation you used to have. You may be resigned to this and feel that your desire for sex has become a lesser priority than other things, like self-discovery, grandchildren, friendship, and travel. Perhaps you've been told that as you age your sexual energy will become directed outward to more spiritual and service-oriented activities.

True, this has been the norm for previous generations, because they did not have the resources to stop the decline in hormones, endorphins, and brain chemicals that keep us looking and feeling sexy. But healthy levels of sexual hormones, equal to those present when we were in our 20s, give us a love for life that can still be directed into both service-oriented activities *and* an active sex life.

Indeed, sexual energy *is* spiritual energy. Sexual energy is the sacred energy of creation, and we certainly can and should enjoy healthy sexuality throughout our lives.

CHAPTER 24

WHAT SURVIVES OF US:
Our Mission for the Next 50 Years

Today's generations are always transforming and defying expectations. Our greatest test is how we handle and redefine aging. How will we live . . . and what will survive of us?

I began writing the first chapter of this book sitting on the white, pristine beaches in Jupiter, Florida. Quite coincidentally, four years later, I find myself back on the same beach to write this last chapter, even though I have moved to California. It's interesting how reflective you become when you sit near the ocean. It is so vast and permanent—an ever-changing witness to millions of years of life. It humbles me, because unlike these ancient waters, our life here on this earth is transient.

Scientists say that approximately 6,000 years ago a great flood occurred and the earth was covered with water. This flooding is depicted in the biblical tale of Noah's ark and in the legends of many other cultures. With the real threat of famine, disease, polluted water and air, infertility, childhood diseases, and on and on, it seems we may once again need a modern "ark" as our means of survival.

We have certainly been made aware of these dangers for some time.

In 1962, a scientist named Rachel Carson wrote a forward-looking and penetrating book called *Silent Spring.* Carson warned us then that human-made chemicals were interfering with the development of our own offspring. She was right. Her book had huge prepublication sales, was serialized in the *New York Times Magazine* prior to publication, and was on the *New York Times* bestseller list for more than 30 weeks. Reaction to its content was loudly and publicly debated. It also inspired a small group of field biologists to begin observing widespread evidence of damage in the birds, fish, and other wildlife throughout the Great Lakes. For their efforts they were reprimanded and given lateral transfers, and their findings were stuffed away in the bottom drawer of a supervisor's desk . . . never published.

Thirty-five years later, Theo Colborn wrote a book that picked up where *Silent Spring* left off—*Our Stolen Future.* She, too, warned us that human-made chemicals interfere with the natural ones that tell our cells, tissues, and organs how to develop and function. In her acceptance speech for the Rachel Carson Leadership Award in 1997 she said:

> Scientists now realize that although effects have been reported in adults who were directly exposed to some of these chemicals, the most sensitive period to exposure occurs prenatally and shortly after birth. The damage is insidious and irreversible and expressed in offspring as inconspicuous loss of function. These are population-wide effects, unlike cancer, acute toxicity, and obvious birth defects. Your children, their children, and all future children are at risk.[1]

It Falls to Us to Change Our Direction

Many of us are finally waking up to the fact that we are heading in the wrong direction and cannot continue on this flawed path any longer. I am quite concerned about the younger generations and *their* future. I am sure you are as well.

Over the course of more than 20 years of training and working in the area of natural foods and healing, I have wondered why we are not doing more to stop the suffering we see around us. For many decades to come, there will be a great deal of pain and heartbreak for all of us, because those who suffer the most will be the younger generations.

So far, we haven't really taken heed of the red flags all around us, yet we still have great potential to reverse our course. Like Noah, let's create an "ark" together and try to save our own families, friends, and the animals we share our planet with. The Body Ecology Way of Life, with its 7 Universal Principles, can be a kind of "ark," guiding us and showing us what we must do to survive these toxic and troubled times.

But how does each one of us give purpose to our time spent here on Earth?

Finding Your Passion

As teens, we asked ourselves questions like *Who am I?* and *Why am I here?* As adults, we are still asking ourselves questions, but they have changed, and we have more of them.

As we grow older, we often wonder: *Who have I become? Will my years spent on this earth have really mattered? I'm here now, but how much time do I have left? Will I leave behind a meaningful legacy? Is there more I need to do?*

Science won't give us the answers to those questions . . . but if we look with our "spiritual eye," the answers become crystal clear.

Each generation has a Universal Purpose. *Each generation brings change. Each of us as an individual* becomes a doorway for change. Each day we have the choice to nourish righteous action so that a superior way of life can be created here on Earth.

Right now we would all agree that the world we live in is changing rapidly around us, and we aren't happy with much of what we see. Yet, many of us are willing to make personal sacrifices to get things back on track. After all, the quality of our own lives, the lives of people we love, and those of future generations depends upon it.

We *will* change . . . because survival is the strongest force in nature, and if we don't change, we humans won't survive. This ocean in front of me will once again be witness to the ending of another civilization.

So, how do you want to use your current interests, skills, and passions to influence the world around you?

About 20 years ago, it began to dawn on me that we were created to serve, and that we are happiest when we are making a difference in the world around us. While you may have purchased this book to learn the secrets to preserving or recapturing your constitutional "prenatal jing," there is an even more deep-seated reason for us to regain or maintain the vibrancy of our youth—we must have the energy, vitality, and mental prowess to transform this planet before we leave. Our future as a human race depends on what we do now!

Indeed, this is why many of us have come. The baby-boomer generation cannot become a burden to the younger generations who will have to care for us if we are no longer able to care for ourselves. Clearly, those of us in my generation must focus our intention on this common purpose, and we cannot leave here satisfied that our lives had purpose until our mission is complete.

Finding Your Tribe

In the past, a tribe was a clan of people who descended from a common ancestor. A tribe today can be defined as a group of people or a "subfamily" that holds common interests or a collective passion. Together they share knowledge and find and implement solutions.

In Seth Godin's book *Tribes,* he talks about how the *individual* has more power than ever before to create change. When people have a shared interest and a shared way of communicating that interest, "miracles" happen. Today's generations are bringing an entirely new business and social-change culture to the world. As Godin says, *heretics* have become the new leaders. These new leaders don't "manage." They connect and inspire. They are not concerned with earnings reports. They are concerned with leveraging skills and resources in ways that make palpable change in suffering lives.[2]

We are a powerful tribe.

With our enormous resources . . . our wisdom, our talents, and our wealth . . . we are more ready than ever to have an intentional and positive impact in the world.

And we are generous.

According to the Corporation for National and Community Service, volunteering in America is at a 30-year high. In fact, the number of Americans volunteering in their communities jumped by 1.6 million in 2009, the largest increase in six years.[3] And the midlife-and-older generations have made more charitable contributions than any other age-group. Our interest in and commitment to volunteerism has resulted in a 37 percent increase in volunteering among midlife Americans since 1989.[4]

What makes the way we give unique? Well, first, we are noticeably more engrossed in making use of our existing expertise and interests, and we want our volunteer activities to reflect our beliefs and what we care about. We have high expectations, want diversity of choice, and tend to bypass opportunities that we don't find interesting or challenging. "Making a difference" is the top reason why we volunteer, and because we see retirement as a new chapter to our lives rather than an ending, we are more upbeat about the future and always on the lookout for ways to stay involved and learn new skills.[5]

Those of us who belong to the younger generations may be even more successful than baby boomers.

Sweeping and transformative change is not something that only midlifers do. More and more universities are changing the focus and curricula of their business programs. Why? Because their students are demanding it! Schools like the University of Maryland have made social entrepreneurship a priority, giving students the opportunity to align entrepreneurial vision and problem solving with philanthropy and social change. (See: **www.rhsmith.umd.edu/svc**.)

We won't follow the sedentary ways of our aging parents, nor will we allow ourselves to become as isolated. Today we are creating new tribes where we can be bonded with passionate members like ourselves—even if they live across a vast ocean—by using technology such as online social networks.

Mother Teresa often said that isolated people are the poorest people on the planet. Don't let loneliness and separation enclose your life as the years fly by. Get involved. Become a member of a tribe that shares *your* passions.

The following is an example of one of my intentions:

Envisioning the "Coffee Shop" the Body Ecology Way— a New Kind of Fast Food

More and more people are working virtually.

Today, as many as one in five employees avail themselves of some type of telework, and this number will only grow as we become more technologically self-sufficient. For the self-employed or the telecommuter, the coffee shop has become an all-important meeting place to network and conduct business. But with the typical coffee shop serving caffeinated beverages and fatty/sweet pastries, what is the health-conscious person supposed to do? Many diets fail because they are by nature "antisocial"—they force people to avoid social situations where unhealthy and fattening food is served. This isolation causes many dieters to feel despondent, which in turn makes them want to eat and return to their old habits! For healthy people today, the coffee shop has become a Catch-22.

In the very near future I envision a chain of "probiotic cafés"—places where people could meet in a more communal setting, socialize, do their work, and eat healthfully at the same time. Instead of a caffeine buzz, customers would enjoy the rush of an herbal tonic made to order—for their unique needs that day—much like they do at Erewhon, one of my favorite health-food stores, located in West Los Angeles. CocoBiotic cocktail or a green smoothie or an anti-aging soup would be standard fare, and so would lots of vegetables, fresh fish and chicken, and of course, grain-like seeds. Wouldn't it be great if you could order your favorite fermented foods as takeout, or enjoy a sugar-free dessert that satisfies the munchies but doesn't pack on the pounds?

What Is Your Passion? Where Is Your Tribe?

Is your passion food? Consider taking a workshop on how to use whole foods to make quick, inexpensive meals. You can pass on what you've learned to your busy children.

Is your passion sustainable agriculture? Join your local Slow Food movement (**www.slowfoodusa.org**), or get involved in your community's farmers' market. If none exists, start one!

Is your passion exercise? Perhaps you will be the person who develops a radical new and fun program to motivate sedentary people to become active and strong so that they are not as prone to injury and illness in their later years.

Is your passion educating children? Why not start a garden at a nearby school or in your community? These local gardens are a great way to get kids outdoors and to teach them about vegetables and other healthy foods. They can actually see the food growing; it helps them make a connection between what's on their plates and where it came from.

Is it your passion to go back to school and learn? I love to learn, and I love to teach. And I am passionate about changing the way the world eats because I know how important this is. I think my greatest love is to teach young women how to create beautiful, healthy babies. I also love giving online classes and teleseminars to explain the Body Ecology Way of Life to anyone and everyone who wants to learn.

Find something that ignites *your* passion and do it. Your chances of being successful are very high, because right now those of us with this positive intention have the Universe (God's Will, or whatever words you chose to use to define your higher power) to support us. So pick your passion, take action, and you will soon see that you are truly making a difference in the world around you. Miraculously, you'll also begin to look and feel much younger. Like alchemy, answers to your personal, health, and financial problems will just also appear—step by step—as you work your own personal touch of magic on the world.

Our Final Chapter—a New Beginning

Imagine what *you* can accomplish when you take care of yourself, as outlined in this book, and then manifest many more decades of life to pursue your dreams. Imagine what each generation will have accomplished as we harmonize our amazing resources!

Never underestimate the power of one person! *You* can make a huge difference in the world—and with social-media outlets such as blogs, Facebook, and Twitter, it has never been easier to do. A new idea or theory, new research, and especially new solutions can find their way around the world in a matter of minutes.

An eternal optimist, I know we can overcome the many challenges facing us, and I am certain that you know this, too. That is why I wrote this book.

I want us *all* to have the energy we need to create a healthier, happier world by serving in the way each of us is trained or is called to do. I wrote this book for *you*. You are alive now; and when you focus on restoring *your* vital energy to serve, you can help herald a shiny, bright new beginning. . . .

Nourish your body and your soul well . . . and when you draw your last breath, you can say to yourself with great pride, *"My life really mattered. I'm glad I came."*

APPENDIX

The Body Ecology Shopping List

Buy organic foods whenever possible.

A sensitivity to any one of the foods in this list, while uncommon, is *not* uncommon when you have digestive problems and immune deficiency. As you create a healthy inner ecosystem, and strengthen your digestion and immune system, you should soon be able to enjoy most of these foods. But remember the Principle of Uniqueness. Find foods that work best for your unique body. We have carefully examined the ingredients in the brand names mentioned below and have given them the Body Ecology stamp of approval ( ). As we learn about new safe and delicious foods and products that help you become even healthier, we will expand and update this list.

ANIMAL PROTEIN

(Free from antibiotics or hormones)
Eggs, from free-range poultry (the best come directly from the
    farmer)
Fish and fish eggs (roe), cold-water, fresh, and frozen

Premium grass-fed ground beef (one supplier we like is White Oak
Pastures [Bluffton, GA], available at Whole Foods and Publix
Markets)
Free-range poultry
Natural beef and turkey hot dogs and sausage (Applegate Farms:
www.applegatefarms.com)

❃

BAKING PRODUCTS

Alcohol-free flavoring extracts
(Frontier: **www.frontiercoop.com**; St. John's Botanicals: **www
.stjohnsbotanicals.com**; and The Spicery Shoppe)
Baking powder (Hain Pure Foods: **www.hainpurefoods.com**)
Pure vanilla powder (Nielsen-Massey Vanillas, Inc.: **www.nielsen
massey.com**)

❃

BUTTER/GHEE

(Preferably from grass-fed cows; many grass-feeding farmers ad-
vertise butter in *Wise Traditions in Food, Farming, and the Healing Arts*, the journal of the Weston A. Price Foundation)
Body Ecology's **Culture Starter** (for homemade cultured butter—
even raw)
X-Factor Gold High-Vitamin Butter Oil (Green Pasture Products:
www.greenpasture.org)
Butter (raw best)
Ghee, also called clarified butter (Purity Farms is organic: **www
.purityfarms.com**)

❃

DAIRY*

(Always best fermented. Visit **www.realmilk.com** for sources near you)

Old Chatham Sheepherding Company (plain flavor) sheep yogurt (**www.blacksheepcheese.com**)

Camel Milk Association camel milk (**www.camelmilkassociation .org**)

Sweetwoods Dairy raw goat's milk (NM: 505-465-2608)

ENZYMES

Body Ecology's **Assist™ Full Spectrum Plant Digestive Enzyme Formula** (for vegetarian meals)

Body Ecology's **Assist Dairy & Protein™** (effectively digests animal-protein meals)

Body Ecology's **Assist SI™** (digests protein, carbs, and fats in small intestines; use at every meal)

FERMENTED FOODS

Body Ecology has starter cultures for making raw cultured vegetables, cultured butter, and sour cream, as well as kefir starter for making traditional milk kefir, young coconut kefir, and kefir cheese. Body Ecology also has fermented probiotic liquids (**InnergyBiotic™, CocoBiotic™, Whole Grains Biotic**, and **Dong Quai™**). Dilute these liquids with sparkling mineral water and they make an ideal replacement for soft drinks when sweetened with Body Ecology's **Stevia Liquid Concentrate.**

Super Spirulina Plus™ (100% fermented protein powder with 50% fermented spirulina) is a very sour, very potent way to nourish your liver, increase iron and magnesium levels, and significantly boost energy. It provides powerful probiotic benefits.

Raw cultured vegetables are now available in many stores around the U.S. There are also private "artisans" who make them and will ship to you. (See **www.bodyecology.com** for listings.)

Raw miso*

Raw natto (no MSG)*

FRUIT

Black-currant juice from Austria (Austria's Finest, Naturally™: **www.austriasfinestnaturally.com**)

Cranberries, fresh or frozen

Cranberry juice concentrate, pure and unsweetened

Lemons, fresh

Limes, fresh

Pomegranate juice or from concentrate

Noni, mangosteen, and açaí juices, unsweetened (Genesis Today™: **www.genesistoday.com**)

GRAIN-LIKE SEEDS

(Remember to soak 8–24 hours)

Amaranth buckwheat (also called kasha)

Cream of Buckwheat cereal (Pocono: **www.poconofoods.com**)

Millet

Puffed Millet Cereal, dry (Arrowhead Mills: **www.arrowhead mills.com**)

Quinoa and Quinoa Flakes (Ancient Harvest: **www.quinoa.net**)

STEVIA, SALT, HERBS, AND SPICES

Stevia: Body Ecology's own great-tasting liquid herbal concentrate with no aftertaste.

Seasoning salts: Herbamare™ and Trocomare™ (A.Vogel: **www.avogel.com**).

Garden herbs (fresh or dried). All traditional land herbs and spices are on The Diet, including antifungal herbs like cinnamon, coriander, curry, garlic, ginger, and turmeric.

Seasonings from the ocean: Maine Coast Sea Seasonings™ Dulse, Dulse with Garlic, Kelp with Cayenne (good substitute for salt and pepper) (**www.seaveg.com**).

Sea salt: The special sea salts we use in our Body Ecology test kitchens are the most medicinal of salts and have a superior "vibrational energy." We recommend you use fine-grind and gray Celtic sea salt for cooking and Hawaiian Makai Pure Sea Salt at the table (Selina Naturally™: **www.SelinaNaturally.com**).

LAND VEGETABLES

All land vegetables except for cooked beets, mung bean sprouts, mushrooms (dried shiitake is okay), parsnips, green peppers, yams, and potatoes (red-skin is okay)

NUTS AND SEEDS

Always soaked and dehydrated

OCEAN VEGETABLES

Agar, arame, dulse, hijiki, kelp, kombu, nori, sea palm, and wakame (Maine Coast™ Sea Vegetables: **www.seaveg.com**; Eden Foods®: **www.edenfoods.com**; and other brands)

ORGANIC, UNREFINED OILS

Extra-virgin olive oil (Rallis™ [**www.rallisoliveoil.com**] has a premium, early-harvest *extra*-extra-virgin oil with a nearly flawless <0.14% acidity—needless to say, it is delicious and our absolute favorite)

Wild Alaskan Sockeye Salmon Oil (Vital Choice™: **www.vital choice.com**)

Coconut oil

Pumpkin-seed oil (Austria's Finest, Naturally™: **www.austrias finestnaturally.com**)

X-Factor Gold High-Vitamin Butter Oil and Blue Ice Fermented Cod Liver Oil (both from Green Pasture: **www.greenpasture .org**)

Fish oil

Flaxseed oil (Barlean's Organic Oils: **www.barleans.com**)

Flax with borage

The Essential Woman or Omega Man (both from Barlean's Organic Oils: **www.barleans.com**)

Macadamia-nut oil

Red-palm oil

SALAD DRESSINGS AND CONDIMENTS

Mustards made with apple-cider vinegar (Tree of Life™'s Whole Grain, Eden™'s mustard, Anne™'s Original Mountain Herb,

Zake™'s Fire Country, True Natural Taste™ organic mustards: 800-559-2998)

Cindy's Kitchen™ Organic Creamy Miso salad dressing (**www .cindyskitchen.com**)

Spectrum® salad dressings (**www.spectrumorganics.com**)

TEAS

(Read labels carefully. There are many great herbal teas available, but green tea is an excellent choice. Avoid teas with citric acid and from fruits like raspberry; raspberry leaf, stem, or root is fine.)

Traditional Medicinals Weightless, Organic Ginger Aid, Organic Mother's Milk, Organic Echinacea Plus, Organic Echinacea Elder, Pau d'Arco, Organic Chamomile, Organic Raspberry Leaf (**www.traditionalmedicinals.com**)

PERSONAL-CARE PRODUCTS

(Antimicrobial)

Thursday Plantation™ Tea Tree Suppositories (**www.thursday plantation.com**)

Tea tree oil castile soap, dental floss, shampoo, mouthwash, and lip balm

NutriBiotic™ Dental Gel (**www.nutribiotic.com**)

Desert Essence™ Natural Tea Tree Oil & Neem Toothpaste (**www .desertessence.com**)

ProSeed™ Feminine Rinse (douche concentrate); ProSeed™ Nail Rescue (antifungal nail formula); ProSeed Healthy Gums

Zion Health ClayBrite Natural Toothpaste™ (**www.zionhealth .com**)

Vita-Myr™ Zinc-Plus Toothpaste (herbal toothpaste with myrrh, clove, and grapefruit seed extract) (**www.vitamyr.com**)

ANTIFUNGAL, ANTIVIRAL, ANTIBACTERIAL IMMUNE BOOSTERS

Oil of oregano
ProSeed Soothing Ear Drops
Olive-leaf extract

SAUNA

Clearlight Sauna (**www.HealwithHeat.com**; 800-317-5070)

OTHER VALUABLE PRODUCTS

Body Ecology's **Vitality SuperGreen™** (preferred to a multi-vitamin, it is designed to help restore your inner ecosystem and supply a wide spectrum of easily digested nutrients)

Body Ecology's **Ocean Plant Extract™** (nourishes the thyroid to increase energy for healing, helps eliminate mercury, and protects against radiation—a must for pregnant women and those with an underactive thyroid)

Body Ecology's **LivAmend™** (helps support a healthy liver, increases bile flow, and improves bowel elimination)

Body Ecology's **Ancient Earth Minerals™** (chelated from ancient plant matter; and an excellent source of energy minerals, trace elements, and amino acids)

Body Ecology's **EcoBloom™** (100% natural chicory extract, a prebiotic to feed friendly flora; can be added to salad dressings, drinks, baked goods, and cultured foods before fermenting)

Genesis Today™'s 4 Fiber (has flaxseeds, hemp seeds, noni fiber, and excellent herbs to promote better elimination; **www .genesistoday.com**)

Lecithin granules (tossed into a salad or salad dressing, this adds creaminess, aids fat metabolism, and is good for the brain and nervous system)

Morningstar Minerals™ Energy Boost 70 (a liquid fulvic acid, chelated from ancient plant matter, it's a great tasteless liquid source of minerals, trace elements, and amino acids that nourish your adrenals and thyroid . . . add to any food or drink you prepare; **www.msminerals.com**)

Morningstar Minerals Vitality Boost HA (great to implant after your colon-cleansing sessions; **www.msminerals.com**)

Xanthan gum (add to salad for thickening)

Irish moss (a great natural thickening agent)

KEFIR PRODUCTS

(Commercially produced are of poor quality and cannot compare to fresh, delicious homemade kefir)

Body Ecology's **Kefir Starter™** (for homemade milk kefir or for fermenting the liquid and spoon-meat of the young coconut)

PROBIOTICS

Your local health-food store carries many excellent probiotic supplements. They all are far more effective when taken with the fermented foods on the Body Ecology program. Our favorite brand is Probulin. It includes not only an inulin prebiotic and well-researched strains of probiotics, but also an acid-protection technology to ensure the safe passage of bacteria through the stomach (**www.bodyecology.com/probulin**).

OTHER BOOKS YOU'LL WANT TO READ

The Body Ecology Diet: Recovering Your Health and Rebuilding Your Immunity, by Donna Gates, with Linda Schatz
The Stevia Cookbook: Cooking with Nature's Calorie-Free Sweetener, by Ray Sahelian, M.D., and Donna Gates

*These foods are not tolerated by everyone. Avoid them the first six weeks, then introduce them by rotating them into your diet once every four days and eat them with alkaline, non-starchy vegetables; avoid eating them alone.

Many of the products listed here are available in your local health-food store. Body Ecology's products (appearing in bold) are available online at **www.bodyecology .com** or by calling 866-4BE-DIET (423-3438). Your local health-food store can also order them for you.

ENDNOTES

Chapter 1

1. Randall Fitzgerald, *The Hundred-Year Lie: How Food and Medicine Are Destroying Your Health* (New York: Penguin Group, 2006): 3.

Chapter 2

1. "Anti-Aging Theories," *New Beauty,* 2004: 70–74.

2. **http://www.antiaging-systems.com/extract/mitochondrial.htm** (accessed 12/1/09).

3. Graham Simpson, M.D., Stephen T. Sinatra, M.D., and Jorge Suarez-Menendez, M.D., *Spa Medicine: Your Gateway to the Ageless Zone* (North Bergen, NJ: Basic Health Publications, 2004): 116.

4. Prof. Serge Jurasunas, "Mitochondria and Cancer," *Townsend Letter,* August/September 2006: 85.

5. "Mitochondria and the Evolution of Human Longevity," as published in *Life Extension,* February 2006, **http://www.lef.org/magazine/mag2006/feb2006_report_mitochondria_01.htm** (accessed 12/1/09).

6. R. F. Loeser, Jr., "Aging cartilage and osteoarthritis—what's the link?" *Science of Aging Knowledge Environment* 29 (2004): e31, as published in *Life Extension,* February 2006, **http://www.lef.org/magazine/mag2006/feb2006_report_mitochondria_01.htm** (accessed 12/1/09).

7. J. L. Wautier and A. M. Schmidt, "Protein glycation: a firm link to endothelial cell dysfunction," *Circulation Research* 3 (2004): 233–238, as published in *Life Extension,* February 2006, **http://www.lef.org/magazine/mag2006/feb2006_report_mitochondria_01.htm** (accessed 12/1/09).

8. J. E. Rofina, K. Singh, A. Skoumalova-Vesela, et al., "Histochemical accumulation of oxidative damage products is associated with Alzheimer-like pathology in the canine," *Amyloid* 2 (2004): 90–100, as published in *Life Extension,* February 2006,

http://www.lef.org/magazine/mag2006/feb2006_report_mitochondria_01 .htm (accessed 12/1/09).

9.   Simpson, Sinatra, and Suarez-Menendez, *Spa Medicine: Your Gateway to the Ageless Zone*: 118.

Chapter 3

1.   Fritjof Capra, *The Turning Point: Science, Society, and the Rising Culture* (New York: Bantam New Age Books, 1982): 253–257.

2.   Nancy Appleton, Ph.D., *The Curse of Louis Pasteur* (Santa Monica, CA: Choice Publications, 1999): 30–32.

3.   Ibid., 34.

4.   "In-Hospital Deaths from Medical Errors at 195,000 per Year, HealthGrades' Study Finds," HealthGrades Press Release, *American Iatrogenic Association,* July 27, 2004, **http://health.groups.yahoo.com/group/iatrogenic/message/1451** (accessed October 19, 2009).

5.   Appleton, *The Curse of Louis Pasteur:* 109.

Chapter 5

1.   Omraam Mikkael Aivanhov, *The Yoga of Nutrition* (Los Angeles: Prosveta U.S.A., 1991): 40.

Chapter 7

1.   Joe Mercola, "Killer Sugar: Suicide with a Spoon," posted January 9, 2009, **http://articles.mercola.com/sites/articles/archive/2000/01/09/killer-sugar-suicide-with-a-spoon-sugar-dangers.aspx** (accessed 12/15/09).

2.   Charlotte Eyre, "Glucose-free increases lifespan, says study," *Decision News Media,* October 3, 2007, **http://www.ap-foodtechnology.com/Publications/Food-BeverageNutrition/ConfectioneryNews.com/Formulation/Glucose-free-increases-lifespan-says-study** (accessed 12/14/09).

3.   Lorraine Heller, "Sugary drinks linked to Alzheimer's, says study," *Decision News Media,* December 10, 2007, **http://www.foodnavigator.com/Science-Nutrition/Sugary-drinks-linked-to-Alzheimer-s-says-study** (accessed 12/15/09).

4.   Fiona Macrae, "Babies hooked on junk food in the womb," *The Daily Mail,* September 28, 2007, **www.dailymail.co.uk/pages/live/articles/health/**

healthmain.html?in_article_id=475375&in_page_id=1774 (accessed 12/14/09).

5.   H. J. Roberts, *Aspartame (NutraSweet®): Is it Safe?* (Philadelphia: Charles Press Publishers, Inc., 1992): 11.

Chapter 8

1.   http://en.wikipedia.org/wiki/Crisco.

2.   Richard Gibson, "Why Trans Fats Are Still Dining Out," *The Wall Street Journal,* June 7, 2006, http://online.wsj.com/article/SB114964917892673457. html?mod=health_hs_research_science (accessed 12/22/09).

Chapter 9

1.   Rob Stein, "Daily Red Meat Raises Chances of Dying Early: Study is First Large Analysis of Link with Overall Health," *The Washington Post,* March 24, 2009: A01.

2.   Thomas Jefferson to Dr. Vine Utley, 21 March 1819. Source: **www.monticello .org/reports/life/vegetarian.html.**

3.   Bess Dawson-Hughes, Susan S. Harris, and Lisa Ceglia, "Alkaline diets favor lean tissue mass in older adults," *The American Journal of Clinical Nutrition,* Vol. 87, No. 3 (2008): 662–665.

Chapter 10

1.   http://en.wikipedia.org/wiki/Popeye (accessed 1/30/10).

2.   http://encyclopedia.vestigatio.com/Spinach (accessed 1/30/10).

3.   Lindsey Tanner, "Study: Vegetables May Keep Brains Young," *The Associated Press,* October 24, 2006, **http://www.washingtonpost.com/wp-dyn/content/ article/2006/10/24/AR2006102401033.html** (accessed 1/30/10).

4.   Sidney MacDonald Baker, M.D., "The Metaphor of an Oceanic Disease," *Integrative Medicine,* Vol. 7, No. 1, February/March 2008.

5.   Susan Owens, in e-mail correspondence with Donna Gates, March 2010.

6.   C. Campieri, M. Campieri, V. Bertuzzi, E. Swennen, D. Matteuzzi, S. Stefoni, F. Pirovano, C. Centi, S. Ulisse, G. Famularo, and C. De Simone, "Reduction of oxaluria after an oral course of lactic acid bacteria at high concentration," Department of Nephrology, S. Orsola University Hospital, Bologna, Italy, PubMed—indexed for MEDLINE, PMID: 11532105.

7. "Genetically Modified Foods are Inherently Unsafe," Institute for Responsible Technology, **http://www.responsibletechnology.org/utility/showArticle/?objectID=212** (accessed 1/30/10).

Chapter 11

1. Karen Hursh Graber, "Mexico's Cooking with Amaranth," **http://www.manataka.org/page1688.html** (accessed 12/20/09).

2. "The Health Benefits of Buckwheat," from *Healthy Reader* website, July 19, 2006, **http://www.healthyreader.com/2006/07/19/the-health-benefits-of-buckwheat/** (accessed 12/20/09).

3. Karen Railey, "Whole Grains: Millet (Gramineae/Poaceoe)," from *Chet Day's Health & Beyond* website, **http://chetday.com/millet.html** (accessed 12/20/09).

4. "Millet," from *The World's Healthiest Foods* website, **http://www.whfoods.com/genpage.php?tname=foodspice&dbid=53** (accessed 12/20/09).

5. Trevor Ellestad, "Quinoa Grain History and Nutrients: Exploring the Origins and Health Benefits of the Mother Grain," July 4, 2007, **http://food-facts.suite101.com/article.cfm/quinoa** (accessed 12/20/09).

6. E. A. Oelke, D. H. Putnam, T. M. Teynor, and E. S. Oplinger, "Quinoa," *Alternative Field Crops Manual,* **http://www.hort.purdue.edu/newcrop/afcm/quinoa.html** (accessed 12/20/09).

Chapter 12

1. Homer, *The Iliad,* translated by Samuel Butler, Book XIV.

2. "Miraculous Messages from Water," from *Water Secrets Revealed* website, **http://www.life-enthusiast.com/twilight/research_emoto.htm** (accessed 2/27/10).

3. F. Batmanghelidj, M.D., *Water for Health, for Healing, for Life* (New York: Warner Books/Time Warner Group, 2003): 25.

4. Stefan Kuprowsky, M.D., "The Body Matrix: Your Key to Health," *Vista Magazine Online,* **http://www.vistamagonline.com/vista_articles/page.php?tp=3&p=1&id=56&s=the_body_matrix_your_key_to_health** (accessed 2/27/10).

5. "Effects of Dehydration," from *Symptoms of Dehydration* website, **www.symptomsofdehydration.com/effects-of-dehydration.htm** (accessed 2/27/10).

6. Batmanghelidj, *Water for Health, for Healing, for Life:* 32–35.

7. Mike Adams, "The Water Cure: An Interview with Dr. Batmanghelidj. Part I—Discovery of the Water Cure," *Natural News,* http://mrgreenbiz.wordpress.com/2009/05/23/the-water-cure-an-interview-with-dr-batmanghelidj (accessed 2/27/10).

8. Stefanie Schoppen, Ana M. Pérez-Granados, Ángeles Carbajal, Pilar Oubiña, Francisco J. Sánchez-Muniz, Juan A. Gómez-Gerique, and M. Pilar Vaquero, "A Sodium-Rich Carbonated Mineral Water Reduces Cardiovascular Risk in Postmenopausal Women," *Journal of Nutrition* 134 (May 2004): 1058–1063, as found on John Briffa, M.D., website, "The health benefits of drinking sparkling (yes, SPARKLING) water," posted January 23, 2005, http://www.drbriffa.com/blog/2005/01/23/sparkling-water (accessed 2/22/10).

9. "Fine Waters Minerality," posted October 2, 2005, on *Fine Waters* website, http://www.finewaters.com/Bottled_Water_Etiquette/Flavor_of_Water/FineWaters_Minerality.asp (accessed 2/22/10).

10. R. Siener, A. Jahnen, and A. Hesse, "Influence of a mineral water rich in calcium, magnesium, and bicarbonate on urine composition and the risk of calcium oxalate crystallization," *European Journal of Clinical Nutrition,* 58 (February 2004): 270–276.

11. Batmanghelidj, *Water for Health, for Healing, for Life:* 227.

12. "Green Tea," from *Silk Road Teas* website, http://www.silkroadteas.com/servlet/the-template/greentea_gateway/Page (accessed 2/22/10).

13. "Pomegranate inhibits hormone-dependent breast cancer cell growth," posted January 8, 2010, on *Life Extension* website, http://www.lef.org/newsletter/2010/0108_Pomegranate-Inhibits-Hormone-Dependent-Breast-Cancer-Cell-Growth.htm?source=eNewsLetter2009Wk51-2&key=Archive&l=0 (accessed 2/22/10).

Chapter 13

1. "Vinegar supplementation lowers glucose and insulin responses and increases satiety after a bread meal in healthy subjects," *European Journal of Clinical Nutrition,* 59 (2005): 983–988, published online June 29, 2005, http://www.nature.com/ejcn/journal/v59/n9/abs/1602197a.html#aff1 (accessed 3/4/10).

2. B. B. Aggarwal and S. Shishodia, "Suppression of the Nuclear Factor-kappaB Activation Pathway by Spice-Derived Phytochemicals: Reasoning for Seasoning," *Annals, New York Academy of Sciences,* 1030 (2004): 434–441, found at http://www.ncbi.nlm.nih.gov/pubmed/15659827 (accessed 3/4/10).

Chapter 15

1. Cedric F. Garland, et al., "Could sunscreens increase melanoma risk?" *American Journal of Public Health,* 82, No. 4 (April 1992): 614–15.

2. *People Against Cancer: Finding the Best Cancer Treatment,* from the *People Against Cancer* website, **http://www.peopleagainstcancer.com/pdfs/ news/20080916n3.pdf** (accessed 10/11/10).

3. Guy B. Mulligan and Angelo Licata, "Taking vitamin D with the largest meal improves absorption and results in higher serum levels of 25-hydroxyvitamin D," *The Journal of Bone and Mineral Research,* Department of Endocrinology, Diabetes, and Metabolism, Cleveland Clinic Foundation, Cleveland, OH, **http://www .jbmr.org/view/0/index.html** (accessed 7/19/10).

Chapter 16

1. Swami Ambikananda Saraswati, *Breathwork* (Hong Kong: HarperCollins Publishers, LTD, 2001): 14.

2. Ibid., 20.

3. Paul G. Harch and Virginia McCullough, *The Oxygen Revolution* (New York: Hatherleigh Press, 2007) 156–174.

Chapter 17

1. Robert Preidt, "Errands Tomorrow? Sleep May Help You Remember," *HealthDay News,* originally published in *Psychological Science,* July 2, 2010, **http://www .medicinenet.com/script/main/art.asp?articlekey=117753** (accessed 7/19/10).

2. *North Carolina Driver's Handbook,* Division of Motor Vehicles, Department of Transportation: 37.

3. F. P. Cappuccio, L. D'Elia, P. Strazzullo, and M. A. Miller, "Sleep Duration and All-Cause Mortality: A Systematic Review and Meta-Analysis of Prospective Studies," *Sleep,* 33 (2010): 585–592, **http://www.journalsleep.org/ViewAbstract .aspx?pid=27780** (accessed 10/6/10).

4. The National Sleep Foundation, "How Much Sleep Do We Really Need?" from the *National Sleep Foundation* website: **http://www.sleepfoundation.org/ article/how-sleep-works/how-much-sleep-do-we-really-need** (accessed 10/14/10).

5. Roni Caryn Rabin, "Behavior: Napping Can Prime the Brain for Learning," *The New York Times,* February 22, 2010, **http://www.nytimes.com/2010/02/23/ health/research/23beha.html?em** (accessed 10/6/10).

6.   Mark Stibich, Ph.D., "Tips for Great Naps," from **About.com** website, December 6, 2008, **http://longevity.about.com/od/sleep/a/napping_tips.htm** (accessed 10/6/10).

Chapter 20

1.   Mikkel Aaland, "Finnish Sauna: History of the Nordic Bath," ©1997, **http://www.cyberbohemia.com/Pages/historyofnordic.htm** (accessed 6/1/10).

2.   "Health Benefits of Saunas," *Doctorline: The Ultimate Directory,* **www.doctorline.com/sauna.htm** (accessed 6/1/10).

3.   Cheryl Richardson, *Take Time for Your Life* (New York: Broadway Books, 1999): 188–189.

Chapter 21

1.   Mary Carmichael, "Strong, Faster, Smarter," *Newsweek,* March 26, 2007: 40–46.

2.   Michael Craig Miller, M.D., "Exercise is a State of Mind," *Newsweek,* March 26, 2007: 48–55.

Chapter 22

1.   Nancy Smith, "Manage Your Stress," from *Real Simple* website, **http://www.realsimple.com/health/mind-mood/stress/manage-stress-10000001550513/index.html** (accessed 10/6/10).

2.   Michelle Andrews, "How to Beat Stress and Angst Through Meditation," *U.S. News & World Report,* December 29, 2008: 2.

3.   Joel Stein, "Just Say Om," *Time,* August 4, 2003: 53.

4.   Ibid., 52.

5.   Peter Kelder, *The Eye of Revelation* (1946), ed. J. W. Watt, Booklocker.com, Inc.: 1st Reprint Edition, January 10, 2008.

Chapter 23

1.   Dr. Dicken Weatherby, *Naturally Raising Your HGH Levels* (Jacksonville, OR: Bear Mountain Publishing, 2005): 1–22.

2.   Ibid.

3. Christine Vestal, "The Science Behind Stem Cell Research," *The Pew Forum on Religion and Public Life,* July 17, 2008, **http://pewforum.org/Science-and-Bioethics/The-Science-Behind-Stem-Cell-Research.aspx** (accessed 10/6/10).

4. "StemCellTherapy21 Launches $15,000 Anti-Aging Therapy with Umbilical Cord Blood Mesenchymal Cells," *PR Log,* July 20, 2009, **http://www.prlog.org/10287130-stemcelltherapy21-launches-15000-antiaging-therapy-with-umbilical-cord-blood-mesenchymal-cells.html** (accessed 10/6/10).

5. Amanda Gardner, "Scientists Find Stem Cells in Hair That Can Become Skin," *HealthDay News/Bloomberg Business Week,* March 11, 2010, **http://www.businessweek.com/lifestyle/content/healthday/636896.html** (accessed 10/6/10).

6. Mohit Joshi, "Human Umbilical Cord Blood Injection Helps Rejuvenate an Aging Brain," **TopNews.in**, March 11, 2008, **http://www.topnews.in/health/human-umbilical-cord-blood-injection-helps-rejuvenate-aging-brain-21412** (accessed 10/6/10).

7. Alexander Y. Maslov, Tara A. Barone, Robert J. Plunkett, and Steven C. Pruitt, "Neural Stem Cell Detection, Characterization, and Age-Related Changes in the Subventricular Zone of Mice," *The Journal of Neuroscience,* 24 (2004): 1726–1733.

8. Al Fin, "Brain Rejuvenation Using Stem Cells From Cord Blood," *Future Blogger,* April 3, 2008, **http://www.memebox.com/futureblogger/show/317-brain-rejuvenation-using-stem-cells-from-cord-blood** (accessed 10/6/10).

9. "Bone Marrow Stem Cell Release Regulated By Brain's Biological Clock," *Science Daily,* February 7, 2008 (reprinted with editorial adaptations by *Science Daily* staff from materials provided by Mount Sinai Medical Center, via *Newswise*), **http://www.sciencedaily.com/releases/2008/02/080206212051.htm** (accessed 10/6/10).

10. "High-Tech Ways to Extend Your Life," **Oprah.com** website, March 24, 2009, **http://www.oprah.com/health/Life-Extension-Technology-and-Tissue-Regeneration/print/1** (accessed 10/6/10).

11. Barbara Kantrowitz, "Sex and the Single Baby Boomer," *Newsweek,* February 20, 2006, **http://www.newsweek.com/2006/02/20/sex-love-the-new-world.html** (accessed 10/6/10).

12. Al Sears, M.D., "Better Blood Flow Where You Need It," *Power for Healthy Living* website, **http://www.alsearsmd.com/better-blood-flow-where-you-need-it** (accessed 10/6/10).

13. Bruce Scali, "Optimal Sexual Health for a Lifetime," *Life Extension,* September 2007: 3.

Chapter 24

1. Theo Colborn, "Acceptance Speech by Theo Colborn Upon Receiving the Rachel Carson Leadership Award," Chatham College, Pittsburgh, PA, June 19, 1997, **http://www.pmac.net/rctc.htm** (accessed 9/14/10).

2. Seth Godin, *Tribes* (New York: The Penguin Group, 2008): 11.

3. Corporation for National & Community Service, Office of Research and Policy Development, *Volunteering in America: 2007 Trends and Rankings in Civic Life* (Washington, D.C., 2007): 1.

4. Corporation for National & Community Service, Office of Research and Policy Development, *Volunteer Growth in America: A Review of Trends Since 1974* (Washington, D.C., 2010): 2.

5. "Great Expectations: Boomers and the Future of Volunteering," *A VolunteerMatch User Study,* MetLife Foundation, 2007.

INDEX

high-protein diets 111
hormonal-decline theory of aging
  11–12
hormone therapy 274–278
hormones
  See also specific hormone
  endocrine system health 85
  hormonal-decline theory of aging
  11–12
HRT 274
human growth hormone (HGH)
  272–273, 274
humanitarian ideals 293–300
hydration 149–171
hydrogenated oils 80, 81
hyperbaric oxygen therapy (HBOT)
  206–209

I

iatrogenic disease 27–28
immunity
  immune boosters, sources 308
  vitamin D 195
individuality *See* Principle of
  Uniqueness
infections, overcoming 34
inflammation
  factors 281, 282
  managing with diet 20, 21
  theory of aging 10, 11
infrared saunas 244
inner ecosystem 21–23, 24
insomnia *See* sleep
insulin
  See also hormones; sugar
  balancing 97
intestines *See* inner ecosystem
iodine 129, 178–179

J

jing 33, 15–19, 253–257
juices *See* beverages

K

kefir
  See also beverages
  milk kefir 61
  starter 98–99
  young coconut kefir 60–61

L

Lakanto 73–74
lamb 98
land vegetables *See* vegetables
laxatives 240–241
leaky gut 30, 119
lipids *See* fats, oils
liver, action of 37
local foods 131
low-fat foods 77–83
lunch ideas 189

M

magnesium and vitamin D 202
margarine 79
massage therapies 260–261
mayonnaise 186
meat
  See also animal proteins
  as protein source 98
  recommendations 99
medical practices, modern 27–28
meditation 261–263
men
  hormone balance 277–278
  sexual performance issues
  286–291
menopause 274–275
microbiota 21–23, 27
milk
  See also dairy
  breast milk 23
  shopping list 302
milk kefir 61, 301

ACKNOWLEDGMENTS

It's just perfect that Hay House is publishing my second book. Louise, your words of encouragement have been in my head for the four years it has taken Lyndi and me to write this book, especially your advice to "keep it positive." Following the Principle of Balance, I've tried to do so, but also wanted Baby Boomers to realize the negative impact our sheer numbers have had on the world, in the hopes that we will take the right steps to correct the problems. When you said you felt that you were "holding a treasure" in your hand, that meant everything to me.

I'm deeply grateful, too, to Lyndi for your insistence on giving this book an almost poetic energy. I know working with a perfectionist is difficult, but I hope you will be eternally proud of what we have accomplished together. Kenneth Storey, you must be the most patient man on the planet. Thank you for making our book beautiful. Carole Addlestone meticulously edited the first part of our manuscript, and when she became too busy, Stephanie Marr did a brilliant job with the second half and with the index. Alex Freemon gave a final polish to everything. Thank you all for your hard, committed work.

I am very fortunate to have an incredible Body Ecology team working with me, helping me bring Body Ecology's message to the world. Without even being asked, they go above and beyond the call of duty, because they believe so much in this work. I can feel confident that you as the reader will find your life enhanced with the information in this book. Please help all of us spread Body Ecology's message; and let's work together to create a happier, healthier world.

I am always deeply grateful to the Force that guides me, opens the right doors, and helps me reach the most amazing people—all who are ready to hear this message.

ABOUT THE AUTHORS

Donna Gates has helped hundreds of thousands of people overcome immune-system disorders and other health issues and achieve peak health. She is known as the teacher to the teachers, and her insights continue to guide many of today's most renowned natural-health physicians and other professionals. An expert on candidiasis (CRC) and related immune disorders, she has done extensive research on how these debilitating conditions affect the body, mind and spirit. She developed and tested the Body Ecology Diet on many different people, who have all improved their health by following the basic principles of The Diet.

Donna is a nutritional consultant, home economist and founder of Body Ecology, Inc., a leading nutrition company. She has studied with the top macrobiotic teachers and graduated from Lima Osawa's cooking academy in Japan. She holds an MEd in Counselling from Loyola University and a BS in Early Childhood Development from the University of Georgia.

Donna is credited with leading some of the most important innovations in natural health, including inventing young coconut kefir, being at the forefront of probiotics and fermented foods, and bringing stevia/reb A (powder and liquid), along with other products, into the United States. She is also the author of *The Body Ecology Diet* (with Linda Schatz).

Lyndi Schrecengost is a professional writer and marketing consultant specializing in health, fitness, education and environmental advocacy. Co-founder of FLUENT Communications, LLC, a Washington, D.C.–based writing firm, she has worked for more than two decades as a communications professional for a wide range of commercial and non-profit clients. Lyndi has a strong interest in all aspects of alternative health and has co-written a number of books on the topic. In addition to *The Baby Boomer Diet,* she is co-writer of *The Genius of Flexibility with Bob Cooley.* She will be assisting Donna Gates on her forthcoming book, *The Body Ecology Approach to Detoxification.* Lyndi holds a BA in Communication Arts, an MA in Literature, and is a graduate of the University of Denver's Publishing Institute. She currently resides in Chapel Hill, North Carolina.

www.bodyecology.com

The Body Ecology Mission

As the leader in fermented foods and nutrition, our mission at BODY ECOLOGY is to change the way the world eats, thus ending disease. We want every home in America to be using the healthy foods we recommend in this book. We want all children to be born with perfect health. With advances in modern genomics coupled with Body Ecology's Seven Universal Principles and our BED foods . . . especially fermented foods . . . this can be our future.

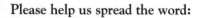

Please help us spread the word:

✔ Eating a variety of cultured foods found all around the world helps create a healthy inner ecosystem and contributes to a long, healthy lifespan.

✔ Organic, unrefined seed oils, coconut oil, extra-virgin olive oil, raw butter, and raw cream are the best fats to eat. Avoid bleached, refined, and deodorized vegetable oils commonly found in most foods. Also avoid margarine.

✔ Stevia is an excellent choice to satisfy your sweet tooth.

✔ Taking an alkaline, mineral-rich superfoods formula is even better than man-made supplements for reversing protein, mineral, and essential fatty acid deficiencies.

✔ Raw apple cider vinegar is the only really healthy vinegar.

✔ Ocean vegetables and organic land vegetables should make up a significant portion of each meal.

✔ Cold-water fish, free-range poultry, and eggs from free-running, fertile chickens are your best sources of animal protein.

BEDROK and Autism

Body Ecology Diet Recovering Our Kids

The Body Ecology Diet (BED), developed by Donna Gates, has been in use for over 15 years to address immune-system issues, including viral and fungal infections, various autoimmune diseases, nutritional deficiencies, and digestive disorders (IBS, ulcerative colitis, and Crohn's disease). For the past several years it has been used experimentally within the autism community with very positive results. BEDROK children improve dramatically when their parents introduce our principles and our foods into their way of life.

The BED views autism as a combination of disorders—all correctable. A gut-brain infection in the early stages of the disorder distances the child from his surroundings. The goal of dietary intervention is to bring him back into our world and back to his true self.

Donna Gates has a passion for helping children. BEDROK (Body Ecology Diet Recovering Our Kids) is a program she is developing together with parents of children with autism. BEDROK has a strong spiritual component to it. Donna truly believes that the children coming into our world today are highly evolved beings and need to be treated as such. She explains, "Our planet is in such turmoil at the moment, and many children in this new generation carry priceless information and solutions to our most serious problems. But these highly evolved souls will come of age unable to fulfill their missions on earth unless we correct the conditions that threaten to hold them back."

Autism has multiple causes, including:

• Undetected infections (fungal and viral)
• Environmental toxins inherited from several previous generations
• Weak endocrine organs (adrenal and thyroid)
• Blocked detoxification pathways that prevent toxins from leaving the body
• Congested livers
• Nutritional deficiencies coupled with vulnerable immune systems due to the lack of an "inner ecosystem"

All these form a complex disorder that takes our children away from us and ultimately will prevent them from accomplishing their spiritual purpose. It is our responsibility to bring them back. The world needs this generation; we can't afford to lose them.

Please visit us at www.bodyecology.com to learn more about Body Ecology Diet research on autism, chat about autism and ADD, and browse a wide range of information and products to recover your inner ecology. Or call 866-4BE-DIET.

Stay Connected with Body Ecology!

You can make a difference in the world by simply joining Body Ecology in its mission to change the way the world eats. The Body Ecology tribe can be found on Facebook and Twitter.

www.facebook.com/bodyecology   BodyEcology

The Body Ecology Facebook fan page is teeming with activity. Great health topics are addressed, and support with helpful suggestions are offered from thousands of health-minded "friends and fans." How can you impact your family, friends, and community? Start living the Body Ecology lifestyle! Learn our system of health and healing, and put it into practice step by step – just watch the difference it will make in your life and in the lives of those around your. Learn more on Facebook and Twitter!

Subscribe to Body Ecology's FREE e-Newsletter

The Body Ecology Health & Wellness e-Newsletter is cherished by readers around the world and widely considered one of THE most important newsletters available. It's an essential read for anyone committed to improving their health. Once you subscribe, you will find health insights and solutions with a strong focus on natural and alternative health angles – long before you read them elsewhere. In fact, many of the world's most renowned and respected natural health physicians and dietary experts have referred to Body Ecology to learn essential insights that are then incorporated into their own health programs and publications.

Even more important, the health and wellness insights you'll discover in every free issue REALLY WORK. The natural/dietary-health-focused articles you'll read are a combination of scientific research, common sense, and factual data. Tens of thousands of people have genuinely seen their health *dramatically improve* through the well-researched and easy-to-understand insights provided by Body Ecology.

Sign up today for FREE at www.BodyEcology.com

We hope you enjoyed this Hay House book. If you'd like
to receive our online catalog featuring additional information
on Hay House books and products, or if you'd like to find out more
about the Hay Foundation, please contact:

Hay House UK, Ltd., 292B Kensal Rd., London W10 5BE
Phone: 0-20-8962-1230 • *Fax:* 0-20-8962-1239
www.hayhouse.co.uk • **www.hayfoundation.org**

Published and distributed in Australia by: Hay House Australia Pty. Ltd.,
18/36 Ralph St., Alexandria NSW 2015 • *Phone:* 612-9669-4299
Fax: 612-9669-4144 • www.hayhouse.com.au

Published and distributed in the United States by:
Hay House, Inc., P.O. Box 5100, Carlsbad, CA 92018-5100
Phone: (760) 431-7695 or (800) 654-5126
Fax: (760) 431-6948 or (800) 650-5115 www.hayhouse.com

Published and distributed in the Republic of South Africa by: Hay House SA (Pty),
Ltd., P.O. Box 990, Witkoppen 2068 • *Phone/Fax:* 27-11-467-8904
www.hayhouse.co.za

Published in India by: Hay House Publishers India, Muskaan Complex, Plot No. 3,
B-2, Vasant Kunj, New Delhi 110 070 • *Phone:* 91-11-4176-1620
Fax: 91-11-4176-1630 • www.hayhouse.co.in

Distributed in Canada by: Raincoast, 9050 Shaughnessy St., Vancouver, B.C.
V6P 6E5 • *Phone:* (604) 323-7100 • *Fax:* (604) 323-2600 • www.raincoast.com

Take Your Soul on a Vacation

Visit **www.HealYourLife.com**® to regroup, recharge,
and reconnect with your own magnificence.
Featuring blogs, mind-body-spirit news, and life-
changing wisdom from Louise Hay and friends.

Visit **www.HealYourLife.com** today!

Free e-newsletters
from Hay House, the Ultimate
Resource for Inspiration

Be the first to know about Hay House's dollar deals, free downloads, special offers, affirmation cards, giveaways, contests, and more!

 Get exclusive excerpts from our latest releases and videos from *Hay House Present Moments*.

 Enjoy uplifting personal stories, how-to articles, and healing advice, along with videos and empowering quotes, within *Heal Your Life*.

 Have an inspirational story to tell and a passion for writing? Sharpen your writing skills with insider tips from *Your Writing Life*.

Sign Up Now!

Get inspired, educate yourself, get a complimentary gift, and share the wisdom!

http://www.hayhouse.com/newsletters.php

Visit www.hayhouse.com to sign up today!